The Vegan Weight Loss Revolution:

Secrets for Lifetime Success

Claudia Rachel Johnsen, Ph.D.

ISBN: 9781702725255

DEDICATION

To all those who want to join
the VEGAN WEIGHT LOSS REVOLUTION
for diet and health,
and to all those who have joined the
VEGAN REVOLUTION already.

To my Mom who was vegan before it was cool.

CONTENTS

ACKNOWLEDGMENTS

Thanks you so much to all those wonderful participants in my
study.

1 A NEW WAY OF DOING THINGS

I stopped eating beef, pork, chicken, fish, egg, and most cheese, and have lost 20 pounds in five months.

The weight loss industry is out to get your money. They may say: "You can lose weight," but what they really mean to say is: "You can lose weight, but you can't do it without us." They want to convince you that the only way to do things is by following their plan. Their plan is the right one after all. They are the only ones that know how to do it. They are the only ones that know what to eat, when to eat, and the exact specifications of food to eat. They say you couldn't possibly be able to figure out just the right amount of protein, the right kinds of fat, how to eliminate carbs, and then even think of having time to cook. They want you to think you need them. Sure, their plans may work, (in fact research shows every diet works for a while) but what they really thrive on is repeat business. How could you possibly keep weight off without their special foods delivered to you?

Well, you know what I think? I think that is terrible! They only want your money and they don't care a smidge about your long-term health or your budget. Weight loss from diet programs to pills to surgery is big business. Just like all the other groups with BIG in their name (BIG Pharma, BIG Chemical, BIG Agra), BIG Weight Loss's purpose is making money for their company and their shareholders by taking money from you. They will come up with their product, make a catch phrase that boosts sales, and they're happy.

But what the weight loss industry is doing is not in your best interest. It is not what research says will keep excess weight off, it is not what research says will prevent yo-yo dieting, and it is by no means what is best for your long-term health. Big Weight Loss wants to tell you it is okay to eat anything you want if it is in small portions. They want to tell a heavy person it is okay to gain weight so they can have their insurance pay for a stomach stapling. Big Weight Loss even says you must swallow their proprietary blend of miracle pills, because you are incapable of doing anything meaningful on your own.

This is a book for the public. This is a book for change. It is my motivation to make you the healthiest you can be. I don't care about politics. I don't care if I'm going to offend some lobbying group or someone is going to pull my advertising. I have no such ties. What I care about is presenting you with accurate information about a very useful, effective weight loss method that just so happens to be great for your health, the environment, and animals, too: Going VEGAN.

This is not a book for researchers. They have ways of getting their information, and frankly they are bought and paid for already, so they have their minds made up. I may be a researcher, but I am far more interested in having you the reader make up your own mind. It is my job to present you with my findings and ask you to give it a go. Constantly debating causes inactivity, both the physical and mental kind. We know what works. We know what is healthiest. It is time to start living the truth. Let us leave the research and the arguing about what should be done up to the researchers and government officials. They are the ones with time to waste.

For myself, I choose action.

<u>"Normal" Isn't Healthy Anymore, It's Time for Something "Radical."</u>

In American we can no longer say "normal weight." Normal weight isn't healthy weight anymore. About two-thirds of Americans are either overweight or obese. It doesn't matter if you don't like those names. That's the medical terminology, and unfortunately, fewer and fewer of us can say that we are a healthy, normal, ideal weight as determined by health outcomes and longevity.

We must stop eating the way we do or those new "normals," the new averages, will keep getting bigger and bigger, and our health as a nation will suffer the consequences. The government's dietary guidelines aren't doing the trick. Fad diets, meal replacements, prescription weight loss drugs, liposuction, and stomach bypasses are not doing the trick either.

This is not the time for spending new money on weight loss pills and mood-altering drugs. This is not the time for lobbying for more "normal-weight" people on TV. The time is over for making excuses. It is time for something that really works.

Could it be that what most of us have been raised to eat our entire lives is doing us harm? Could it be that some of the basic components of our diet are making us heavier and heavier? Have you ever felt like you were the only one who couldn't figure out how to eat less, or count calories, or eat less fat? Why does something so natural as eating seem to be so difficult? Why is it that others don't seem to be affected by foods in the same way you do? Could it be that you are not alone? I am here to tell you, "You are not alone." The American diet is failing us. The animal product laden, chemically processed diet of today is not doing us any favors.

I truly believe, we are the masters of our own destiny. You are the only one that knows how you feel both physically and mentally. You are the only one that can take charge of what you consume and determine how you feel when you eat. No one else can be inside your skin and experience your exact experiences. But we are all human, we share the same basics, and we can learn from others who have had similar problems and gotten over them. We can listen to them, see what worked for them, and try what they tried to see if it might work for us, too.

I am a researcher. I like studying research articles, but I also like seeing what works in real life. This book is about the experiences of one hundred fifty-one individuals who made it work. It is about individuals just like you who tried multiple times to lose weight. It is about what they tried and what worked. It is about their feelings and triumphs. It is about their mastery over their diets, their weight, and their life by taking a few simple steps to eliminate animal products from their lives.

If you wanted to build a successful business, you would get advice from someone who had a successful business. If you wanted to make a million dollars in the stock market, you would follow the strategies of a multimillion-dollar stock investor. So, if you want to lose weight, you look at people who did so successfully. The key that is different here is not that these people lost weight. We've all done that before. The key is that they were able to keep it off for good and get healthier in the process. It is very hard to get good results on any experiment for any length of time. However, people in this study had continued success for over ten years by following a vegan diet.

Maybe it is what we have been conditioned to eat that is truly strange and radical. Maybe it is time for a fundamental change in just what we think is food.

How to Use this Book

It is hard for me to tell you how to use this book. Some people want to start a diet right away. Some people want to be convinced that a diet will work before they give it a try. Some people want to know what others did and how they felt before they give it a go. Others want to come to the root of their thinking and understand themselves to see if changes might work for them. She might love getting on a scale and he might hate measuring his waist. You might love to think about all the things you will gain if you lose weight, but you also may be more motivated by thinking of all the things you might lose if you don't. This book has it all. So please feel free to read it in order or jump around as you see fit. It's all good!

<u>Serious Symptoms to Address Before You Start</u>
There are many known outcomes to carrying excess weight. Some relate to physical health. Some relate to your mental health. Some relate to your social health.

Right now, we are going to focus on your physical health.

I am extremely serious about this next part. I want you to put this book down, stop everything else you are doing, and call your physician right now if you experience any of these symptoms:

- Pain in your chest, neck, or jaw,
- Pressure or squeezing in your chest,
- Shortness of breath at rest or relaxation,
- Dizziness,
- Fainting,
- Swollen ankles (edema),
- Difficulty breathing when you are lying down,
- Shortness of breath or coughing when lying down or sleeping,
- Feeling like you are having rapid, hard, or abnormal heart beats,
- Feeling like you are having irregular heartbeats,
- Aching, crampy, tired, or burning pain in the legs, or
- Unusual shortness of breath or fatigue while doing your normal activities.

These are all major signs and symptoms of disease and need to be addressed by you physician.

If you are experiencing any of these, you need to call your doctor. And I will emphasize, you should not do any type of exercise program if you are experiencing any of these. You need to be evaluated by a physician so both of you know what is going on with your current state of health. Keep these symptoms in mind and if you experience any of them, contact your doctor.

I will give you similar lists throughout this book based on different health conditions. Keep in mind that if you have any of these symptoms now or in the past, talk to your doctor. Remember, your doctor doesn't know everything, especially if you don't tell him or her. By learning about the symptoms of various health conditions, in this case conditions related to excess weight, you can alert your health care providers to symptoms that should be addressed and might have been overlooked otherwise. In my book, the best cure is prevention.

Also, if you smoke, you are automatically considered at high risk for health problems and should be evaluated by a physician before starting any new diet or exercise plan.

The above symptoms can be signs of coronary artery disease, hypertension, problems with glucose metabolism, high cholesterol levels, and other serious health problems. If you experience any of these, or are experiencing any other worrisome signs or symptoms, call you doctor and get it checked out. It is always better to be safe than sorry. Only after you have had these problems addressed by your own physician should you address changes in your diet and exercise.

<u>An Action Plan to Understanding and Doing Something about Weight Loss.</u>

Okay, you're overweight. You're too heavy, chubby, obese, big-boned, or whatever you want to call it. We could be nasty and call you all kinds of names. We could be nice and say you have a pretty face. Whatever it is though, you know it and you know it is wrong. But it is not who you are, and it is not what you want to be. You have tried tons of things and for whatever reason, they haven't worked, or they worked for a while and you gave up. Perhaps you were so happy you achieved your goal weight that this was the end of all the willpower you could muster, and that was it, and your weight went back up.

Maybe we have been listening to the wrong people. Now

that I think about it, of all the nutritionists I've known in my many years of education, work, and teaching, most were overweight, if not darned right obese. Just about all those researchers and all those counselors have the very same problem that the average Joe has. They are too fat. Maybe that is because they eat just like everybody else. They know all kinds of things, but they are stuck in their heads. In fact, they can't even agree what a healthy diet is. All they want to do is argue and debate. By the time these scientists figure it all out, we'll all be dead.

To give them a little sympathy though, this is a very hard thing knowing what a healthy diet is. Everyone is different, and everyone is an expert. It doesn't matter how much you have studied. Everyone is an expert because they know what they like to eat.

I am an expert in nutrition, but I'm not an expert in what you like. I can't follow you around and feed you and make all your meals for you. Your mother can't even do that anymore. So, I'm going to teach you what science knows about weight loss, and let you decide, and experiment, and find out what is right for you. Only by finding what is right for you, will you come to be happy and healthy.

Now, first off, if weight loss was so easy, and scientists, dietitians, and doctors knew everything, then we would all be lean and beautiful. Our food supply would also be vastly different. If you haven't figured out by now though, our food supply is not based on what is healthy. But scientists and government officials don't know everything, and they can't even agree. They just see the problems and complain. They can't take action because that would be too upsetting for the public and for their pocketbooks, especially if it means promoting a vegan diet.

But I can tell you what they do agree on. They agree on what happens to you if you stay overweight, that is, what diseases you are likely to get if you stay overweight. But don't think they mind and don't mistake this for caring. They are perfectly willing to push you the next pill because it is their mission to "take care of" you.

So, when you are trying to motivate someone, you have two approaches: the carrot and the stick, that is, the reward and the punishment. If you are like most people, you are much more likely to be motivated to avoid the punishment than you are to seek out the reward. You can picture yourself lean and beautiful all you want, and that is fine, but is that all you need to motivate yourself, and stay motivated? For most the answer is no. If it was, this probably would not be the umpteenth book on diet that you have read. Most people just say they weren't born that way, or they were thin when they were younger. But I believe that we can all be healthy and beautiful, since we were all made that way. Something in our environment is failing us.

So, let's try the stick approach for a moment. This is the same approach that dog owners who use shock collars for barking and electric fences use. The dog gets shocked, cruelly. Now, I'm not advocating this, and I wouldn't do this to my own pet. However, we can use the same approach with ourselves. No, we are not going to shock ourselves physically, but we will hopefully shock ourselves mentally and motivate ourselves into permanent change. That change in our thoughts needs to be a drastic reconsideration of everything in order to have an effect. If we do not shock ourselves enough, there will be no reason to question something so basic and fundamental about ourselves as what we eat. Why would we ever admit what we like is wrong?

For most people, this mental shock comes when they go to the doctor's office for a physical, or maybe when they are trying to buy life insurance, and they get bad news. There are different levels of this bad news. Maybe you're told you have high blood pressure let's say. Now that is a shock, but maybe that is not a very big shock and the doctor puts you on medication. He or she tells you that you're one of millions of Americans with high blood pressure, gives you a few things to try, and sends you on your merry way. You don't feel too bad leaving the office. After all, we're all getting older and it is just one of those things.

Now, let's try another scenario. This time you go to the doctor, and he or she tells you that you have inoperable cancer that has spread everywhere, there is absolutely nothing you can do, you will suffer immensely, you have at most a month to live, and it will be torture until the very end. Without a doubt, you would be absolutely devastated. Perhaps you might want to kill yourself. You would try anything or give anything for some ray of hope. If you heard there was one doctor on the planet that could help you, and that doctor was on the other side of the world, you might cash in your life savings to get a plane ticket to get to this physician and pay for the treatment for at least a shot at staying alive.

Well, first, I hope that you are not sick with anything, even the slightest cold. Second, as the insurance agents will tell you, if you're not suffering any ill effects of your excess weight, the odds are that you will, if not now, you will sometime in the future. It is my hope that that diagnosis will be a slight one, like our high blood pressure example, and not a catastrophic one, like our cancer example. However, let's use our stick approach for the next several minutes to examine what is most likely the outcome of excess weight.

These are the conditions that you can count on for your future if you are obese. Roll the dice and bet on these: inflammation; diabetes; cardiovascular disease including coronary heart disease, hypertension, atrial fibrillation, and stroke; chronic renal disease; cancer including leukemia, multiple myeloma, non-Hodgkin's lymphoma, and cancer of the endometrium, esophagus, kidney, breast, colon, and rectum; osteoarthritis including chronic pain and disability; nonalcoholic fatty liver disease; insomnia and obstructive sleep apnea with short sleep duration, impaired sleep quality, and irregular sleep patterns; gallbladder disease; and mental health issues including major depressive disorder.[1]

---

[1] Steelman, G. Michael. Health Hazards of Obesity. ," Obesity: Evaluation and Treatment Essentials, Second Edition. G. Michael Steelman, Eric C. Westman, eds. CRC Press, New York, 2016.

What would life be like dealing with these? Perhaps it is worth trying a radical dietary change if it means avoiding these.

Later on, in this book, we will do mental exercises to help us visualize the awful possibility of these and help us condition ourselves to never let them happen.

The future is not written in stone. We can change our weight and our health for the better. Knowing how to mentally condition yourself for success is one of the key factors that people who have lost weight and kept it off know how to do. But for now, let's start with the most significant thing you can change to positively affect your health and lose weight:

Your Diet.

CHAPTER 1

A NEW WAY OF DOING THINGS

SUMMARY

- The Big Weight Loss is out to get your money. They want repeat business and don't really care about your health.
- If we want to learn how to do something, we should try to learn from someone who has done it already.
- A vegan diet is a healthy, lasting solution to weight loss and health.
- We can change how we feel about food.
- We should address any possible health conditions with our doctor before proceeding.

2 THE DIET

I lost 25 pounds in 5 months becoming a complete vegetarian.

What Kind of Diet is This?

You know we are talking about going vegan. Wait a minute, before you discount this idea all together, you don't have to go cold turkey. You can take things slowly, but the rewards you can see are measurable and great. I am judging from the fact that you even have this book in your hands, that you are open to the idea.

Let me tell you a bit about the benefits.

One, it means weight loss. It sounds simple enough and it really is. Eliminate those foods that are the culprits to keeping you heavy.

If you look at average serving sizes for various types of foods, those with the most calories are meat, dairy product, eggs, and animal fats. Have you ever thought of eating a lot of fruits, vegetables, and whole grains to make you gain weight? No, of course not. (Well, maybe you could say dried fruit and pastries, but we'll get into that later.)

For the most part if you look at foods of animal origin compared to foods of plant origin, the foods that have the most calories are of animal origin. Here, is why: Animal products contain more fat, and fat has more calories per gram than either protein or carbohydrates. While carbohydrates and proteins contain 4 calories per gram, fat has over double – 9 calories per gram. That is, in the same amount of space, fat has more than twice as many calories.

Think of it this way: Remember the School House Rock song that went: "A gram is about the size of a raisin, about the same as a paperclip. Now isn't that amazing?" So, you can think of it in terms of size. You can eat double the amount of food in carbohydrate and protein than you can in fat and have the same number of calories. So, what would be more fun: Eating lots of tasty foods or only a few tasty foods? If you love to eat, like me, I opt for eating more. And what is the way to do that? Eating foods low in fat.

"Wait a minute!" you say. "I tried that low-fat thing and I didn't work."

That's right. Much of America did it, too, but they didn't do it in a way that was also low sugar and processed, white foods. When the food industry heard that they had to do the low-fat thing for marketing, they thought: "There goes taste!" So their solution to makeup for it was to pump-up the sugar, salt, processed grains, and chemicals. So like everybody else, it didn't matter that the food was low in fat, we ate a ton of it because they made it so tasty! Too tasty!

But if you eat lots of highly processed foods, you miss out on the nutrient packed goodness of whole foods, that satisfy you in a low-calorie way.

If you take mice and feed them a healthy mouse-food diet and let them eat as much as they want, the mice eat until they are full and that's that. They eat what they want, are satisfied, and are a normal weight. But if you take rats and feed them what we might call "junk foods," or as some other researchers call "the supermarket diet" or a "tasty diet," as much as they want, they eat and eat, and turn out to be obese.[2] Just like most

---

[2] Anthon Sclafani, Deleri Springer. Dietary obesity in adult rats:

of us did! They can't control themselves when the food is super-process and super-tasty, and neither can we. They used to say that children up to five years old could determine just what they needed to eat to grow and maintain their weight. They used to teach counselors to tell moms, "You provide the food and let them determine how much they want to eat." Unfortunately, you can't really say that anymore. The food supply has changed so much that we all eat too much. We see this in the skyrocketing number of obese children. They will suffer just like us, but at an earlier age, all the problems associated with obesity.

But, more about the low processed, low sugar foods later. The other thing you will note from these relatively old studies (1976) is that the supermarket-fed rats reject bitter foods. These bitter foods, like green vegetables are often some of the best foods for us. They also worked less to obtain food. Plus, they did not increase their activity levels to compensate for the increased caloric intake.

This sounds just like us, doesn't it? Junky food makes us reject food that is good for us, put less effort into getting food thus going for the convenience food, and get sluggish and lazy.

The food we eat must be healthy to make us feel healthy. Eating junk is going to make us feel like junk.

If you are going to eat a low-fat, lower-calorie diet, which actual is a great way to lose weight, what then is the easiest, healthiest way to do so? One might be to read every label for how many calories and how much fat foods have, memorize the content of foods, and carry around a pocket calorie and fat guide and perhaps a food scale, and count calories. Another, I believe, easier way is to simply eliminate the major high-fat and high-calorie culprit foods, namely animal products.

Becoming vegetarian, and working your way to vegan, means a lot of other great things, too. The diet we are talking about is the healthiest diet there is. I mean it for everybody.

Similarities to hypothalamic and human obesity syndromes. Physiology & Behavior. Volume 17, Issue 3, September 1976, Pages 461-471.

What other diet is there that cuts down on disease, helps you live longer, and helps the planet along the way as well? You would be hard pressed to find a diet with as many benefits as vegetarianism/veganism. (I say both for now because there are few research studies exclusively on veganism.) Well, we will talk more about those reasons later. For now, on with the weight loss!

But What About Protein?

People say a lot of critical, disbelieving things when you say you don't eat meat. I think maybe the most common one is, "Where to you get your protein?" This is a great question, especially in these days of high-protein, Atkins-style weight loss diets. In a way, it does make sense to eat lots of protein if you are trying to lose weight. After all, protein has about half the calories of fat and the same number of calories as carbohydrates. But, high-protein diets don't make sense. Here is why:

Many problems have been reported with high-protein diets. These include loss of energy, constipation, bad breath, difficulty concentrating, gallbladder problems, heart problems, reduced kidney function, kidney stones, elevated cholesterol, gout, and osteoporosis.[3] In fact the Medical Research Council of the British government has condemned high-protein diets because of their association with kidney damage and the Norfolk and Norwich Hospital in England has banned them.[4]

While people may lose weight on a high protein diet, the diet is not sustainable since most people feel so poorly. Even more bad news is that when they go off the diet to any degree, they not only gain back the same weight, but they gain back more weight than they previously lost. That is, they get heavier. They would have been better off not going on a diet in the first place than struggling and feeling poorly. To make matters worse, more of what they gain back is fat than it previously

---

[3] "Low Carb, High Risk," <u>Good Medicine</u>. The Physicians Committee for Responsible Medicine. Winter 2004, Vol. XIII, Num. 1.
[4] Ibid.

was. So, they are fatter and unhealthier.

My grandmother, who was born in 1910, was put on a no-meat, low-salt diet when she was very young for kidney problems. That was maybe 1920. My point is that science has known for a very long time that meat and salt are bad for the kidneys. High-protein diets are high in the branch chain amino acids, leucine, isoleucine, and valine. These amino acids are basically shaped like a "V" and they tend to get stuck in the kidneys.

Kidney problems are not the only thing though. Heart problems can also result or be worsened on a high-protein diet. In November 2003, the Physicians Committee for Responsible Medicine held a news conference at the Press Club in Washington, D.C. There physicians and former high-protein diet followers described the health risks associated with high-protein, low-carbohydrate diets. Participants included the relative of a sixteen-year-old who died after developing a heart arrhythmia which developed while on a high-protein diet. They also included relatives of a forty-one-year-old man who died of a sudden heart attach also while on a high-protein diet.[5]

One major problem is pre-existing kidney disease. In general, since those with chronic kidney disease often do not know they have this condition and since high-protein diets can be so detrimental, it has been recommended that all individuals "undergo a screening for serum creatine and a urinary dipstick test for proteinuria (protein in the urine)" before starting such a diet.[6]

Dr. Allon N. Friedman states: "High protein consumption has been found, under various conditions, to lead to glomerular hyperfiltration and hyperemia (over filtration by the kidneys and increased blood flow to the kidneys); acceleration

---

[5] "Atkins Dieters Report Serious Health Problems," <u>Good Medicine</u>. The Physicians Committee for Responsible Medicine. Winter 2004, Vol. XIII, Num. 1.

[6] Allon N.Friedman MD. High-protein diets: Potential effects on the kidney in renal health and disease. American Journal of Kidney Diseases. Volume 44, Issue 6, December 2004, Pages 950-962.

of chronic kidney disease; increased proteinuria (protein in the urine); diuresis (excessive urine production), natriuresis (excessive sodium in the urine), and kaliuresis (excessive potassium in the urine) with associated blood pressure changes; increased risk for nephrolithiasis (the formation of kidney stones); and various metabolic alterations."[7]

These problems are not part and parcel of a vegan diet. You can get plenty of protein on a vegan diet. We will discuss specifically later on. But for now please note that as long as you eat a variety of foods, a vegetarian (progressing toward vegan) diet is nutrient rich including protein. So feel free to start cutting out all meats from your diet as soon as possible to help get you started on your road to weight loss.

<u>Notes on the Meaning of Vegetarian and Vegan?</u>
These words mean different things to different people. People might say they are vegetarian meaning they don't eat meat. But then if you ask them further, they might have meat when they are out to dinner or get BBQ. Indeed, the word "meat" might mean red meat to some, and beef, pork, lamb, poultry, fish, shellfish, etc. to others. Some people may call this flexitarian (eating vegan sometimes) lately. Some vegetarians may drink milk. Some may eat eggs. Some may eat cheese but not drink milk. Some may not eat eggs and yet have them in baked goods. Some may call themselves vegan or pure vegetarian and others may not.

All of this matters more to researchers like me than to most. The one thing you should take away from this discussion though is, that for the purposes of weight loss, the more you eliminate all animal products from your diet the more ideal your weight should become. It doesn't matter what you decide to call yourself.

There are some caveats to this, however. For instance, I don't want you stopping all animal products and replacing them with sugar cookies, potato chips, and diet soda. They

---

[7] Ibid.

might be vegan, but if that is all you eat you probably will not be healthy nor a good ambassador for a vegan diet and this book.

Using this book as a guide you can lose weight, in a healthy way, while eliminating, all at once or gradually, all those unhealthy products from your diet. Keep an open mind. Weight loss is a journey and a key component of it, I believe, is loving yourself and others along the way. Be kind to yourself and others, and try not to make a fuss over semantics.

What Makes for a Successful Diet?

The secrets in this book make for a successful diet. Not all diets are successful as far as I am concerned. These are my criteria for a successful diet.

A successful weight loss diet must:

1. Help achieve weight loss.
2. Be healthy.
3. Be maintainable.
4. Be the healthiest diet for longevity.
5. Be abundant, not restrictive.
6. Not create health problems.
7. Not require medical supervision (in most cases).

Did you know that any weight loss diet you go on generally works? On just about any diet, most people will lose about twelve pounds. Sounds great, right? This one is not a big deal. For most of us, if we lost weight once, we pretty much know how to do it again. It is the other criteria where different diets fall short.

Second, a successful diet must be healthy both in the short-term and in the long-term. While the diet we ate to lose weight may have worked, it may not be healthy to stay on long-term. This is exemplified by the recent studies on decreased longevity associated with high-protein and ketogenic diets.[8]

---

[8] Sara B Seidelmann, MD, Brian Claggett, PhD, Susan Cheng, MD, Mir

The authors state that, "low carbohydrate dietary patterns favoring animal-derived protein and fat sources, from sources such as lamb, beef, pork, and chicken, were associated with higher mortality, whereas those that favored plant-derived protein and fat intake, from sources such as vegetables, nuts, peanut butter, and whole-grain breads, were associated with lower mortality."[9] Since I would like to live as long as I can, and would like you to as well, let's stick to my "vegetables, nuts, peanut butter, and whole-grain breads."

My third criteria states that a successful diet is maintainable. There is no sense eating one way to lose weight and then "going off the program" and gaining it back. Studies show that weight fluctuations are detrimental to health. Better to keep the weight off. Right? This is perhaps why Weight Watchers changed their logo to "WW." Sounds like they want us eating their prescribed "wellness" program forever. But, wouldn't it be great just to eat and not have everything come from the company store? Fluctuation in body weight can have negative health effects that are independent of obesity and being overweight. Those whose weight fluctuated have a higher risk of coronary heart disease and death than those whose weight stays stable.[10]

Fourth, the diet should be the best for promoting health and therefore longevity. Why not eat a diet as close to the healthiest as possible? If we need to lose weight, it is often for our health. Since we are trying to be healthier, why not increase our lifespan as much as we can? Does anyone ever say that

---

Henglin, BA, Amil Shah, MD, Lyn M Steffen, PhD, Aaron R Folsom, MD, Eric B Rimm, ScD, Walter C Willett, MD, Scott D Solomon, MD. Dietary carbohydrate intake and mortality: a prospective cohort study and meta-analysis. The Lancet. VOLUME 3, ISSUE 9, PE419-E428, September 01, 2018.

[9] Ibid.

[10] Lauren Lissner, Ph.D., Patricia M. Odell, Ph.D., Ralph B. D'Agostino, Ph.D., Joseph Stokes, III, M.D., Bernard E. Kreger, M.D., Albert J. Belanger, M.A., and Kelly D. Brownell, Ph.D. Variability of Body Weight and Health Outcomes in the Framingham Population. June 27, 1991. N Engl J Med 1991; 324:1839-1844.

they don't want to see their kids get married and meet their grandchildren? A vegan diet is the basis for longevity.

Fifth, the diets should make you feel there are many foods to eat and you are not being deprived. A successful diet makes you feel like there are an abundance of foods and does not make you feel restricted. If you have gotten this far, I am sure that you are ready for the abundance of new foods, recipes, and flavors that your new lifestyle will open you to. People will ask you, "Do you miss eating meat?" And you will want to reply, "I don't give it a second thought. There are plenty of delicious foods to eat. In fact, I'm trying foods and recipes I never even knew about before I went vegan."

Sixth, successful diets don't create health problems. Severe caloric restriction or reliance on just a few foods can cause serious health problems. There are very few things that you can do to make the diet in this book unhealthy, and we will discuss those later. But I guarantee you that any of these little obstacles are nothing compared to the major pitfalls of the diet you have been on before, the Standard American Diet.

Seventh and lastly, in general, no medical supervision is needed while on this diet (and when it is, I'll tell you). Other diets, such as ketogenic or very-low-calorie diets, bariatric surgery, or pharmacotherapy (pills) require ongoing physicals, blood work, adjustments to medications, and the addition of medications to counteract the side effects caused by other medications or surgeries. Trying to get healthier should not create more medical problems. Most people report general improvement in their health as they eliminate animal products.

Like any other diet, everyone is going to tell you to have a physical. You should have a physical yearly anyway. You should also have a physical before you start any new exercise program. The more overweight you are, the more important this is. You may think you are healthy, but the likelihood is that the heavier you are, the greater your chance of comorbidities. That is, the greater the change of other health problems or diseases existing at the same time as being overweight. So, get your physical and find out what you physician says, but for most people our plan is not going to require ongoing medical supervision, and the expense that goes with it.

Potential Bias

We all have our share of bias. You may have dismissed anything in this book and not even picked it up because you think that vegetarians are crazy, and vegans are even crazier. But, I am glad that you have an open mind and are willing to make changes for your health. I'm not going to tell you that you don't have to change or that you can change for a while and then give up.

Everyone is looking for an easy way out. You may feel a little deprived when you make changes in your life, but later I will give you lots of "mental" exercises to help you feel great about your decision to become healthier. These mental exercises are the kind of thing that builds resilience and make you a stronger person in all aspects of your life.

Resolve today to start making your diet healthier.

Qualitative Research.

The type of study results I am presenting are from a qualitative study. That is, I'm not going to tell you how many pounds you will lose when you become vegetarian or vegan based on your current height and weight, or anything like that. I haven't taken a group of people and made them become vegan for any length of time and studied their metabolism, blood, exercise levels, etc. In other words, I haven't taken real people and put them in a box and made them the subjects of my laboratory experiment.

Real people, in the real world, don't do well sticking to any program unless they have real motivation to do so. Also, real people don't like living in a laboratory and having everything they do monitored. So how is a qualitative study different and useful then?

When you do qualitative research, you examine peoples' experiences and what they say. You look for what they did, why they did it, how they felt, and what worked for them. You can then report on questions pertaining to who, what, when, where, why, and how something happened. You can look at their motivations, their family relationships, or any other factors that they report. That is, the researcher may never have thought a factor was important to participant's success, yet there it is in the research as put forward by the participants as being a key factor. From this data, the researcher then can then study further the possible modes of action for the study having the results it did. The possible mechanisms why a vegetarian/vegan diet can aid in weight loss are quite plausible. These mechanisms can then be studied further. Here are some reasons why a vegan diet works:

<u>Mechanisms of Action of a Vegetarian/Vegan Diet for Weight Loss.</u>

So why would becoming a vegetarian/vegan expedite weight loss? These are some possible ways it might work:

1. A vegetarian/vegan diet contains fewer calories than a standard American diet. Any time you eat fewer calories, you lose weight.
2. Most vegetarian/vegan foods are less caloric dense than nonvegetarian foods. The less caloric density, the fewer overall calories are consumed. Plus they take up more space and make you feel more satisfied and full.
3. The more meats, dairy, and eggs are eliminated, the more caloric dense foods are eliminated from the diet.
4. People become more conscious of their overall diet as they eliminate animal foods. Most people who become vegetarian/vegan take a new interest in food, where it comes from, how it is processed, and how healthy it may or may not be. They start reading labels more. Because of this, the overall diet tends to become a healthier one. Less sugar is used.
5. A vegetarian/vegan diet is more nutrient dense, while being less caloric dense. That is, you don't need to eat as many calories to get as many nutrients. We'll talk about specifics of this later. But for now, think of it

this way: Your body knows it needs specific nutrients and will crave them, thus making you hungry, until your requirements are satisfied.

6. A vegetarian/vegan diet includes less appetite stimulators, both naturally occurring and man-made. By sticking to natural foods, appetite stimulating substances that make you want to eat and cause you to eat more, are diminished and fewer calories can be consumed. More on this later, too.

7. A vegetarian/vegan diet contains more fiber and other substances that make you feel fuller longer.

<u>What the Research Results Reveal.</u>
Analysis of my research with 151 participants who made the transition toward veganism shows the following, that you can do, too:

1. People lost weight on a vegetarian diet. The more meats they ate before starting the diet, the more they lost when they stopped eating them.

2. People lost additional weight when they became vegan. For most people, this was more weight than they had initially lost than by cutting out meats alone. It all depended on how much they ate to begin with. For example, people who ate a lot of dairy, lost a lot when they stopped eating it.

3. People gained back weight when they added back meats, eggs, or dairy to their diets. People who added back some meat generally did so only on occasion and discontinued it again when they were able to notice detriments to their health and/or weight regain. These connections to their health often only became apparent when they added these foods again. People regained weight when they added eggs and dairy to their diets again. Most people eliminated these foods when they noticed weight gain or other health concerns. The more weight people had lost when they initially discontinued eggs and dairy, the more likely

they were to eliminate these foods from their diets again.

4. People saw a large, rapid initial weight loss when they eliminated meat, eggs, and dairy from their diets. This was larger the further their weight was away from a healthy, ideal weight.

5. People's weight stabilized at or close to a healthy, ideal weight after this initial weight loss.

6. People maintained their weight loss. The longer it had been since the initial changes in their diet and the more they adhered to their new diet, the better, and longer lasting their results.

7. Lastly, and perhaps most importantly, participants practiced specific motivational techniques that kept them on their diets and changed their outlook on life so that they never wanted to return to their former state. I will teach you these so you can keep the results you earn, too!

<u>Let's Talk about the Results.</u>

One hundred fifty-one (151) people responded to my notices in various health and diet magazines for people who lost weight when they became vegetarian. They lost an average of 36 ½ pounds each! This ranged from ten (10) pounds to 155 pounds. It took an average of seven (7) months to see this weight loss at an average of 1 1/3 pounds weight lost per month. Participants saw significant weight loss in as little as a month, with larger amounts of weight loss occurring, as desired, for as much as three years.

Participants lost an average of 20 percent of their initial body weight. This ranged from six (6) percent of initial body weight to 54 percent of their initial body weight. Successful weight loss as defined by the medical profession of ten (10) percent of initial body weight is considered successful. To lose an average of just under twenty (20) percent of initial body weight is highly significant and really shows the likelihood of success.

Successful weight lost is defined by the medical profession as keeping the weight lost off for one year. Some of the participants in my study were in the middle of their weight loss experience, so you cannot get at this figure for everyone. However, participants reported being able to keep the weight off for an average of 7 ½ years and all those who responded to my follow-up survey (sent out ten years after the initial study) were able to keep the weight off for the full ten years. Participants, who had lost all the weight that they desired, reported keeping it off between one and 33 years.

A Note on Study Design.
If you want to know if a certain substance has an effect, there are different ways that you could determine the answer. You could take that substance and expose it to cells in the laboratory. Using such a method you would have two groups, one that is exposed to the substance in question and the other which is not exposed to the substance in question. This second group is needed and serves as the control. The other group, which is exposed, is called the case or experimental group. Thus, this is a case-control experiment. This is the kind of experiment that researchers look at to "prove" causation. They come up with such statements as: "this chemical causes cancer." However, this only shows that this is true under the circumstances that the scientist used for their experiment, that is, these cells in a laboratory.

You could expose laboratory animals to see what results you get. This kind of experiment introduces all kinds of variables that were not in the first experiment. Whole living things are much more complicated than cells in a dish. You now have additional problems to solve such as what kind of animal do you use, what do they eat, are they sick or under stress, etc. In the laboratory, again you take two groups, an experimental group and a control. If you are careful, in a laboratory you can control just about everything, and in this way, again, you can prove causation. However, this again is only causation under the circumstances that you established in the laboratory. How you attempt to get around this is by repeating your experiment over and over again to get the same results. What researchers then attempt to do is extrapolate their results to humans. For most things, especially diet, I believe this does not work. For this reason, among others, I am against animal testing.

Most researchers you talk to say that this type of case-control study is the strongest proof. That is, it shows causation. I, however, believe that this does not truly represent how the human body works in terms of diet. Humans are extraordinarily complex, much more than any other animal, and they are pretty darn complex, too. We have all kinds of social, economic, cultural, biological, health, mental, and other constraints upon us, not to mention we have very long lives, much longer than any animal we look at in the laboratory. If you put people in a study regarding diet, there is only so much you can control. We could put people in a laboratory (which indeed has been done) and control everything they eat and do. But when you try to do a study on a free-living population, there is only so much you can do, and only so much you can measure. Just figuring out how much someone ate is tricky. Usually, people will report that they eat less than they do, and it is hard to get anyone to stick to a program for a long period of time. For this reason, I prefer to look at epidemiological studies.

Epidemiologists look at the relation between diseases (and health) in populations. These are the kind of studies that the National Geographic Blue Zone researchers looked at to determine the longest living populations in the world. By looking at groups that have the characteristics in question, we can see the long-term relationships between various health outcomes, diet, and lifestyle. These Blue Zone groups with the longest life-spans in the world are predominantly vegetarian and include the Seventh Day Adventist community of Loma Linda, California.

My point in all this is three-fold. One, vegetarian/vegan lifestyles are related to long-term health and longevity. Two, you are what you do most of the time. Long-term health is not about taking a pill. It is not about trying veganism once. It is not about eating something "healthy" once a day, and then eating crap the rest of the day. It is not about eating what you want and taking a pill to make-up for it. It is not about eating a gluten-free food that is really junk in disguise. It is about eating a healthy diet and having a healthy lifestyle most days of your life. It is about being happy with what you eat and being happy in general. You are made up of what you have been eating for years, not just what you ate yesterday. And three, study results need not be on cells, animals, or humans in an artificial setting with artificial parameters to be valid. People live in real life and study results from real life are valid.

The good news is the eliminating animal products works for both weight loss and health. Weight loss will take time, just as gaining weight took time. You will have your good days and bad, just like before, but this time you will know with conviction that you are doing something that is healthy, long-term, that you can live with for life. You will know that what you are doing worked for others and that it is a healthy, long-term life-style with lasting results. Through the course of this book, you will be able to customize your diet to feel your best and help yourself make the best you possible.

<u>Why This Diet Works.</u>

My study shows that vegetarian diets are effective for weight loss. By consuming less caloric dense, higher nutrient dense foods, participants were able to eat less calories and lose weight. Their bodies got what they needed without excessive calories. Most health care professionals will tell you that in order to lose weight, you must expend more calories than you consume. Changing to a vegetarian diet can accomplish this goal. It is my belief that the elimination of meats (all meats including cow, pig, chicken, fish, etc.) is much easier to maintain, and understand, than trying to figure out how many calories, what size portion, difference cooking methods, frequency of consumption, day-to-day variations, binges, etc.

make on the intake of meats and their relation to weight. It is easier to cut them out altogether.

My research also shows that those who adhered to a vegan diet saw additional weight loss in proportion to the percentage these products were in their previous diets. The more milk, cheese, eggs, butter, etc. they ate initially, the greater the weight loss when they discontinued them. Again, the total elimination of these foods appears to be easier than trying to figure out which of these foods are still allowable and just how much.

Now you may say, "Sure they lost weight they gave up a huge part of their diet and didn't know what to eat and were starving themselves until they figured out what to eat instead." Yes, this could be, but there are plenty of meat and milk alternatives. Secondly, it is very difficult to maintain a caloric deficit of even 100-200 calories a day (what doctors say is needed to lose weight) without compensating somewhere. There is something about a vegan diet than allows the consumer to be nourished and satisfied. Perhaps it is its high volume. Perhaps it is its high nutrient content.

Bariatricians (doctors who do stomach surgery for obesity) consider a 10 percent weight loss maintained for one year to be a success. That means if you weighed 300 pounds, lost 30 pounds, and kept it off for a year, you are considered a success. So much for you if you are still 270 pounds! You will see from my results that some participants lost well over this, even 100 pounds, and kept the weight off for years.

It is standard thinking that someone who lost large amounts of weight, and wants to keep it off, needs to exercise 60 to 90 minutes almost every day of the week to maintain these results. Participants report, however, that a vegan diet can greatly reduce these exercise requirements. (Exercise is not physical activity. Physical activity is moving around. Exercise is done expressly for fitness. I enjoy both, but personally don't have that much time to spend. I don't know about you.) Many of the study participants who lost large quantities of weight did not exercise the so-called required hour to an hour and a half a day.

Certainly, you may lose weight if you don't know what to eat, but this does not seem to be the cause of weight loss in my results. Most people reported that they were very happy learning new recipes and trying new foods.

Several people reported that when they added back certain nonvegan products, for whatever reason, their weight went up. Again, nonvegan foods are for the most part higher calorie. The interesting thing about this though is that these same people noticed the reappearance of health problems that they had not previously attributed to their diets. Becoming vegetarian, and then vegan, is what allergists call a type of elimination diet. In an elimination diet, you go on a very allergy-free diet and then add back foods, one at a time, to see if there are any symptoms when they are introduced. This is essentially what these folks did on their own and often decided to eliminate these foods again because of the detrimental effects they had on their weight and/or health.

Most people in my results saw a large initial weight loss. Certainly, this kept them motivated. However, a large initial weight loss on a ketogenic, high-protein diet may indicate cause for concern. Indeed, rapid weight loss is often an indicator of illness. The people in my study felt good though and their weight stabilized at a new, healthy set point. (More on set-point later, but for now know that it can be very difficult for the body to adjust to a new set point. Your body really wants to bounce back to its old weight, that is, the weight that had been too heavy for you.) Somehow, the body knew this new weight and this new diet were healthy, and it didn't have to fight to maintain its fat stores. In other words, it didn't think you were experiencing a famine and didn't panic to hold on to adipose tissue and make you eat in excess.

What is so different about a vegan diet for weight loss is the extraordinary level to which people maintained their weight loss. This is not a yo-yo diet. This is not having to buy pre-packaged calorie-controlled meals for the rest of your life. Because this is not a diet in the traditional sense of the word, but a lifestyle, it is about finding a diet that is right for you, one that is healthy, and you can maintain for the rest of your life.

Now some people think that they cannot live without their meat or milk, and we will make sure you understand all of your nutritional needs later in the book, and there are certainly lots of reasons for becoming a vegetarian or vegan. But purely as a method for weight loss, a vegetarian progressing toward vegan diet is a highly effective, safe choice.

It fits all my criteria for a successful weight loss plan:

1. Weight loss.
2. Health.
3. Maintainable.
4. The healthiest for longevity.
5. Abundant, not restrictive.
6. Does not create health problems.
7. No medical supervision is required in most cases.

Perhaps the most important result of this research though has not been stated yet. It is this: *Participants practiced specific motivational techniques that kept them on their diets and changed their outlook on life.*

I call this "something only we know." It isn't really, but those vegetarian and vegan crusaders are certainly good at it!

<u>The Mind Secrets of Veggies.</u>
The reason why most people know important health and diet information and don't follow it is very simple. They haven't conditioned these things into their brain and behaviors. They haven't made it part of their personality. They haven't internalized these traits and feelings. They haven't made the information meaningful and personal enough. They haven't engrained it in their psyche so much that if they go against it, their actions would go so much against their deep-seated feelings of themselves, their worth, and their values that it would be revolting to them and might make them physically ill.

In essence, they have changed at the root of their being what they consider to be food.

I want you to not only know how to lose the extra weight that you want to get rid of and be healthy, but I want you to keep it off and be healthy and happy the rest of your life. This takes changing how you think. I'm not saying there is anything wrong with how you think now, just, if you are not happy with your weight and your health how you currently are thinking affects your actions and it is up to you to change things if that is what you decide. It is your personal responsibility to take charge of how you think, and you have the ability to first decide to change, and then take action.

Guess what? Vegetarians time and time again, in study after study, live longer than the general population. I want you to internalize what they know and be healthy and happy forever.

I am going to show you how to do this permanently.

When you deal with belief and feelings, as all food consumption ultimately is, you need to look at the psyche. I am going to give you exercises throughout this book to help you examine your own psyche when it comes to your diet and your health. Please do these exercises to your own ability and with your own discretion.

Let me tell you what I mean by this. I have several relatives who died recently. If I tried to do any mental exercise that related to their deaths and my own health, this may be very upsetting. It might be all right, but I may not want to do it in a setting with people I didn't know or even a friend. My husband might be the only one I'm comfortable sharing my true feelings with.

When it comes to my weight, I may not necessarily want to share those feelings with my husband either. It could lead to tears, just like exploring my feelings concerning death, but I know I would feel stupid crying. Still, these are my feeling and I may want to do these exercises on my own. Everyone is going to have a different set of circumstances, and everyone's feelings are equally valid. Getting to the root of your emotions (good or bad), and your feelings and emotional connections concerning food can go a long way towards producing long lasting change.

Let me give you an example of how this might work:

You're a kid that loves animals. You read a book about how animals are exploited by humans for all sorts of things from big game hunting to dog fighting, from battery egg cages to slaughterhouses, and animal testing on mice to psychology experiments on monkeys. The author is very good. Of course, he wants you to feel the animals' plight and he is very graphic in his descriptions. Afterall, he is writing to persuade you that animals are indeed harmed and wants you to take on his opinions and take action. Now, you could read this book any number of ways. You could read it without any emotion just as facts or you could really take matters to heart and cry bitterly as you read or anywhere in between. Let's say the author after all this detailed information said that one of the biggest things you could do to help animals is to become vegan? Who do you think would become vegan and stick to it the most: the person who read it in a detached, unemotional way or the kid who loved animals that read it with emotion and feeling? Certainly, you're the kid who loves animals and took things to heart. You let the book affect your soul. You let the book change your life. And you became vegan and stuck with it!

I am sure there are tons of people who fit this scenario. There were some in my study in fact that became vegan for animal rights and lost weight as an added, wanted benefit. Vegetarian/vegan authors can be very good at this type of thing and I suggest if you have any inclination to read any books on any of the many heartfelt reasons to become vegetarian or vegan, please do so. The more you take these matters to heart, the greater your convictions will be. And it doesn't really matter what reason you stick to your new, healthier diet, the result will be the same. The more you take things to heart the better your compliance with the goals you will set for yourself and your weight loss.

Reading books that give various reasons to be vegetarian or vegan can help you do what you want; that is, change what you think is food. And sometimes it is easier to do thinks for others than it is for yourself. I urge you to explore vegetarian and vegan philosophy books on everything from the environment to animal rights to religion. What these books do not do though is give you specific mental exercise about the health consequences of excess weight. That is what you will find here in Chapter 4: RECLAIMING YOUR HEALTH PHYSICALLY & MENTALLY. Using these exercises can have the same effect of conditioning yourself mentally to change what you consider is food and fit for your consumption because of its effects on your health and the impact that your health has on those around you. The more you put these ideas into practice, the more you will know "The Mind Secrets of Vegetarians."

<u>Tastes do Change.</u>
So, I know you are already open-minded about your diet. If you weren't, you probably would not have a copy of this book in your hands. If you are feeling nervous or upset about the possibility of giving up some of your favorite foods, I want you to know this: People's tastes do change.

The food marketing giants have the general public hooked on fat, sugar, and salt. We are so hooked in fact, that if we have less of these, we can't taste them anymore. We say it needs salt, or it needs some butter, or maybe it's not sweet enough.

For fat, people who are used to eating deep fried foods, butter, or the like have a tolerance for one hundred percent fat. People who eat chips or pretzels, for instance, have a very high tolerance for salt and can almost eat that straight, too, like fat.

Sugar has what they call a "bliss point" which is different for certain groups of people and ages. This is that perfect point that is just right for sweetness (usually quite high) as it is paired with other food. Most people will not eat straight sugar. It is the pairing with other ingredients that makes it most pleasurable. Some of those other ingredients are also other sweeteners, with slightly different tastes, that make the product have a different "depth of flavor" since those other sweeteners react to the taste buds (and brain) in slightly different ways. Also, young children like their sweets tart or sour more than adults do. That is why tart candies are marketed toward kids and chocolates toward middle-aged women.

Salt, sugar, and fat (along with a slew of chemicals) also make the cost of producing these products cheaper for the producer. In fact, apart from adding water or air, salt, fat, and sugar are the cheapest way to bulk up food, and thus reduce the cost. In fact, one of the functions of sugar in the food science/food manufacturing lingo is as a "bulking agent." It costs little and takes up space. Unfortunately, for us though, it packs in the calories, has little other nutritional value, and makes us want to eat more, both because it is stimulating (like a before dinner aperitif drink or an appetizer) and not satiating (satisfying).

The good news though is that your tastes can and do change. As you cut down on salt, sugar, and fat you can taste the other flavors more clearly and everything just doesn't taste of salt, sweet, or fat. These tastes change as you cut out animal product consumption as well. Meat is usually very salty. Who would eat a steak without salt after all? The chef judges on TV say you didn't "season" it properly if you don't add salt and pepper. Meat is also usually very fatty. What is bacon without dripping fat? Dairy products are sweet, first from the milk sugar (lactose) naturally in the dairy, and secondly from added sugar (think "fruit" yogurts). They may also be high in fat and salty such as cheese. Salt is used in making the cheese and regular dairy is fatty. Salt, sugar, and fat sell. Don't be fooled by big business, low-fat dairy doesn't sell without some added sweetener.

Becoming a vegetarian can dramatically reduce your fat intake. Becoming vegan can further cut down your fat intake, but you will also cut down your salt and sugar intake as well. And the more you want to be a healthy veggie, the more you will find yourself cutting down on these appetite-stimulating, calorie-excessive salty, sugary, and fatty foods.

Very many of the respondents to my study said that they no longer craved salt, sugar, and fat. They often reported that the foods that were once their favorite, they now couldn't stand. One woman said this about her once favorite doughnuts:

"I loved them (doughnuts), but I can't imagine ingesting such a disgusting thing now —white flour, sugar, and rancid oil."

Funny, hey?

Scientific studies back this up, too.

Decreasing the salt in your diet reduces the amount of salt that you find pleasant in food. Studies show that after a period on a low-sodium diet, "the preferred level of salt in food is dependent on the level of salt consumed and this preferred level can be lowered after a reduction in sodium intake."[11] That is, the less salt you eat, the less salt you like and the more you can taste it.

As for fat, "consuming a low-fat diet increases the ability to perceive small differences in the fat content (of foods.) Consumption of a high-fat diet significantly decreases taste sensitivity among lean subjects but does not in overweight and obese persons."[12] So, the authors conclude, if you are on a low-fat diet, you can taste when you are eating something that is too fatty. However, on a high-fat diet, lean people can taste when something is fattier, but heavy people could not tell the difference.[13] That tells me two things: One, if you want to know if something is fatty, better to have it on occasion rather than always eating a fatty diet, and two, if you are overweight, your ability to taste can be impaired. Again, your tastes can change toward liking lower fat foods as well. Part of this increased taste sensitivity may indeed come with weight loss.

As for sugar, again, tastes do change. In one study, after one or two months on a low-sugar diet, participants rated low-

---

[11] Bertino, M et al. "Long-Term Reduction In Dietary Sodium Alters The Taste Of Salt." The American Journal Of Clinical Nutrition, vol 36, no. 6, 1982, pp. 1134-1144. Oxford University Press (OUP), doi:10.1093/ajcn/36.6.1134.

[12] Stewart, J E, and R S J Keast. "Recent Fat Intake Modulates Fat Taste Sensitivity In Lean And Overweight Subjects". International Journal Of Obesity, vol 36, no. 6, 2011, pp. 834-842. Springer Nature, doi:10.1038/ijo.2011.155.

[13] At least in this study.

sucrose samples of pudding as more intense than those not on a low-sugar diet. The same effect was found for sweetness in beverages, but with not as strong an effect.[14] You've probably heard that if you eat calories, you can tell you've eaten them. However, if you drink your calories, you can't tell, and you're still hungry. This study bears this out. We can't tell as well when drinks are sweet. You can add a lot of calories with sweetened beverages. Cutting them out of your diet (or strictly limiting them) is a great way to cut down on excessive calories. Kids in particular can really gulp down the sweet drinks. This includes soda and juice. Soda certainly is not needed, and juice, if you are relying on it for vitamin C really can be limited. A half to three-quarters of a cup of orange juice will have you covered. Anyway, a vegan diet usually has loads of vitamin C, so even that may not be needed.

Back to another detriment of sugar. Sugar can actually make you hungry. After being given something sweet, people will have a greater appetite.[15] This is especially true with the artificial sweeteners aspartame, acesulfame potassium, and saccharin which will not only make you hungry, but hungrier than if you had sugar instead.[16] [17] "Aspartame has the most pronounced effect of these, possibly because it does not have a bitter aftertaste. Unlike glucose or sucrose, which decreased the energy intake at a test meal, (eating aspartame first) had no effect."[18] This suggests that while natural sweeteners may make

---

[14] Wise, Paul M et al. "Reduced Dietary Intake Of Simple Sugars Alters Perceived Sweet Taste Intensity But Not Perceived Pleasantness". The American Journal Of Clinical Nutrition, vol 103, no. 1, 2015, pp. 50-60. Oxford University Press (OUP), doi:10.3945/ajcn.115.112300.

[15] Black RM, Leiter LA, Anderson GH. Consuming aspartame with and without taste: differential effects on appetite and food intake of young adult males. Physiol Behav. 1993;53:459–466.

[16] Blundell JE, Hill AJ. Paradoxical effects of an intense sweetener (aspartame) on appetite. Lancet. 1986;1:1092–1093.

[17] Rogers PJ, Carlyle JA, Hill AJ, Blundell JE. Uncoupling sweet taste and calories: comparison of the effects of glucose and three intense sweeteners on hunger and food intake. Physiol Behav. 1988;43:547–552.

[18] Ibid.

it hard for you to keep your overall calorie intake the same, artificial sweeteners definitely make it much more difficult.[19] This is why a lot of researchers blame increased rates of obesity on the increased consumption of artificial sweeteners. Obesity has gone up as artificial sweetener consumption has risen. So, the take home message is: You may wind-up eating more with artificial sweeteners. So instead of trying to replace sugar with something else, just try eating less sweets for a while, and your tastes will change.

Now, I'm not saying that a vegetarian or vegan diet can't contain salt, fat, and sugar. It certainly can. As you start to eliminate animal products from your diet though, most people will naturally cut down on a lot on the unhealthy levels of salt, fat, and sugar. But, don't worry. You can still have fun eating. We are just going to make it a lot healthier.

<u>Putting Things in Action.</u>
This is not a sit back and do nothing but read book. We are going to do specific things to get our weight and health in order.

So, let's start!

<u>Incorporating Inspiration</u>
Most people when they go on a diet head off like gang-busters in the beginning. It is easy when things are new. You are already an expert on diet. Like everybody else, you know what you like to eat. You've researched many diets. You've lost weight multiple times. You may have been on Nutrisystem or whatever else and you've been a repeat customer. You know how to do it.

But there is a difference between losing weight and keeping it off, number one. There is also a difference between eating what will make you lose weight in the short term and living a

---

[19] Yang Q. Gain weight by "going diet?" Artificial sweeteners and the neurobiology of sugar cravings: Neuroscience 2010. Yale J Biol Med. 2010 Jun;83(2):101-8.

long, healthy life, number two. This is where most people need help.

The two main things most people need are:

One, motivation.

And, two, knowledge about what specific components of our diets result in longevity. It's just good that longevity is related to a healthy weight. That means you don't have to even be skinny, if you don't want to.

I frankly would rather live a long life and be healthy and happy, than miserable and sick. I also happen to care greatly about other people. That's what makes you lucky. Yes, I have a doctorate in nutrition, and I can spout all the studies to tell you why you should do such and such. But my work is also interdisciplinary. That means I have researched many topics and have many tools for helping you maintain your motivation, which is really the hardest thing for achieving and maintaining the weight you desire.

Did she say, "You desire?"

I sure did. You are the master of your destiny. You are the one that gets to decide. You are the one that decides when you eat and what. I'm not going to follow you around and feed you or cook for you. I'm not your mom. I've got my own kids and I don't even do that anymore with them. They're not infants anymore and neither are you. Even with kids, you can't force them to eat. You put the food in front of them and they decide what to eat. But there is good news if you have members of your household that should lose weight, too. The person that does the most shopping in the household is the gatekeeper and the one to decide what the other family members eat, most of the time. So, if that's you, and even if it is not, you can profoundly influence the health, and potentially the weight, of the other members of your household.

So, if you picked up this book, my guess is that you are dissatisfied with yourself. Most likely you are dissatisfied with your weight, but your probably dissatisfied with other things about yourself, too.

So, here is the first thing we are going to do. Yes, you have to do somethings for this book. You are not just going to read through it and expect it to work, are you? This is part of the motivation we all need help with. So, let's take it step by step. After all, you are not just what you ate yesterday. You are literally made of what you ate over the course of your entire life, plus a little magic pixy dust your parents and the powers-that-be threw in. So, here is the first step.

<u>Mental Exercise: How to Lose Weight.</u>
As we said before, I know you are an expert in weight loss.

And that is just it. You are the expert in your own weight loss and maintenance of a healthy weight.

You know what you are capable of. Don't be shy. This is your book. Research shows that the more you write things down, the more likely you are to remember them and act on them. (By the way, handwriting improves your memory more than typing, so take all the notes you want and have fun brainstorming!)

Write here, or in another notebook if you like, write ten different things you have heard or tried to do to lose weight:

1)

2)

3)

4)

5)

6)

7)

8)

9)

10)

Please write your ideas down before looking at mine. Your ideas are probably superior to mine.

Here are some ideas for losing weight:

- Eat vegetables.
- Drink water.
- Use smaller plates.
- Use tall glasses instead of fat glasses.
- Make your own soda with seltzer and juice.
- Drinks lots of water.
- Eat less salt, sugar, and fat.
- Eat whole grains.
- Don't stuff yourself.
- Get a good night's sleep.
- Don't rush your meals. Take your time and chew.
- Eat fruit.
- And you thought I was going to say go vegan right away, didn't you? Of course, this is a great idea, but let's get into that a bit later. Let's start with talking about and getting our motivation up first.

Did you like any of these ideas? If so, go back and make a star next to the one you want to start right now. It doesn't matter if it was your idea or mine. Just pick one and commit to making it part of your life from now on.

Yes, I did say from now on. Unfortunately, if you have been overweight for some time, the longer you are at that weight, the body tends to consider that weight normal. Scientists call this your set weight or set point. If you want to lose weight and keep that weight off, you need to establish a new set weight. That means you need to think of this as the first day of the rest of your life. You must be reborn, as it were, and make yourself anew. Pick one idea of yours or mine, and make it yours from now on. If you didn't like the ones you wrote down initially, think of another one that you feel you will have great success in keeping.

You will notice that I did not write down, "Don't eat this and don't eat that." "Dieting" tends to be punitive. After all, "diet" contains the word "die." This is not a punishment. I don't want you to feel bad about eating things and then feel you must punish yourself with diet and starvation later.

Achieving your ideal weight is just that. An achievement!

We live in a society of excess. Excess food, excess turmoil, excess excitement. Maintaining health can be very difficult. Eating too much, or smoking, or doing drugs, or yelling at your family are the easy way out. They are the common, easy things to do. But that is not what you are going to do. You are an extraordinary person, destined to do what only you can do! And you deserve health and happiness, including a healthy weight.

So, if you put all kinds of things in your list of ideas of what you shouldn't do, e.g. "Don't eat this and that," try to think of some things you could do that are fun and positive instead. Maybe it would be fun to make you own sodas with juice and seltzer for instance. Maybe you could try something new every time you see something new in the produce section of the grocery store. Whatever it is, pick something you want to do and make it happen!

<u>Photo Exercise: What You Eat.</u>
Throughout this book I will give you motivational tools you can use to keep you on track. Your cell phone can be used as a highly motivational tool.

If you like to take pictures, you're just like me! And a lot of other people, too!

My father took pictures of everything and he had stacks and stacks of photos. I used to, too.

But now we are lucky ducks. We've got our cameras right on our phones. I thought things were easy when I got a digital camera! Cell phone cameras are so much better. Don't you think?

So, here is a creative assignment:

Start taking photos of everything you eat. Frankly, a lot of people are doing this anyway to post the pretty things they eat on line and promote various restaurants or foods. But instead of taking pictures of just what you think is pretty, or what the waiter brought, take pictures of everything you eat.

Make it fun. Most of us carry our cell phones around everywhere, so you have everything you need. Take pictures of the food in the box. Take pictures of the box. Take pictures of the label including the ingredients and the "Nutrition Fact" label. Take pictures of the food on your plate. Try and get pictures of everything you eat and drink. Post the pictures online and try and make a little money with them, too, if you want. What the heck? You might as well.

Make it as fun as you can, you photography buff!

Now why are we doing this?

Right now, it is just for fun, but later in this book you can use those photos for some mind games and some deep thinking. Those pictures are going to become your record and your tool for a new you.

You can start by taking photos of everything you eat in a single day. Then look back and think to yourself that this is the amount of food that I need to eat to be this weight. Think to yourself: "Is this the weight I want to be? If not, this is not the kind or amount of food that I want to eat. I can do better." When you look at the amount of food you eat in an entire day, it will make a bigger impression than when you just look at each meal or snack. All those foods add up. As you change your diet, you will then be more visually able to see both the kinds of food and the amounts of food change as your body changes.

<u>More on the Diet.</u>

The vegan diet is a highly nutritious, nutrient dense, extremely healthy diet. It may be different than what you are used to eating, but frankly, that is the point. Think about what you have eaten your entire life. Has it gotten you to a point in your life and an appearance that you want? Vegan diets are associated with lower body mass indices (BMIs) even in populations that normally experience more obesity.[20]

Randomized clinical control trials show that a vegan diet has significantly more weight loss than a meat-eating, fish-eating, or semi-vegetarian diet[21] which is the same thing found in my study as well. If you want to lose more weight, the more you go towards a vegan diet the better. Vegans also lower their total fat intake and the intake of saturated fats, thus helping weight loss and improving their risk of disease.[22] These results play out long-term in other studies with significantly more weight-loss than other "more conventional" diets.[23] These results play out even when portion sizes are not limited.[24] Studies show that the consumption of meat is related to weight gain even when you take into account the total energy consumed, that is, you can eat the same number of calories as a vegetarian, but if you eat meat, you will gain more weight. This plays out for red meat, chicken and other poultry, pork, and processed meat.[25]

---

[20] Singh PN, Jaceldo-Siegl K, Shih W, Collado , Le LT, Silguero K, Estevez D, Jordan M, Flores H, Hayes-Bautista DE, McCarthy WJ . Plant-Based Diets Are Associated With Lower Adiposity Levels Among Hispanic/Latino Adults in the Adventist Multi-Ethnic Nutrition (AMEN) Study. Front Nutr. 2019 Apr 9;6:34.

[21] Turner-McGrievy GM, Davidson CR, Wingard EE, Wilcox S, Frongillo EA. Comparative effectiveness of plant-based diets for weight loss: a randomized controlled trial of five different diets. Nutrition. 2015 Feb;31(2):350-8.

[22] Ibid.

[23] Turner-McGrievy GM1, Barnard ND, Scialli AR. A two-year randomized weight loss trial comparing a vegan diet to a more moderate low-fat diet. Obesity (Silver Spring). 2007 Sep;15(9):2276-81.

[24] Barnard ND1, Scialli AR, Turner-McGrievy G, Lanou AJ, Glass J. The effects of a low-fat, plant-based dietary intervention on body weight, metabolism, and insulin sensitivity. Am J Med. 2005 Sep;118(9):991-7.

[25] Vergnaud AC1, Norat T, Romaguera D, Mouw T, May AM, Travier N,

Clinical trials have shown that a low-fat vegan diet decreases your intake of saturated fat and trans fats, while increasing your polyunsaturated fat intake including the essential healthy linoleic fatty acids and alpha-linolenic fatty acids. This in turn decreases the amount of body fat and improves insulin secretion.[26] That is great news for both weight loss and diabetes. Even when comparing women of the same normal BMI levels (similar weight to height ratios), vegans have lower body fat percentages. This is amazing when you consider that the comparison groups in this study all had similar calorie, total fat, and carbohydrate intakes.[27] This is contrary to what most weight loss experts will tell you. The mantra is that a calorie is a calorie, and that if you eat less or exercise more, you will lose weight. Perhaps though this is not the case. I'm here to tell you what you eat makes the biggest difference, especially in the long term. Vegans eat more fiber and more total polyunsaturated fatty acids and omega-3 fatty acids. So, forget the fish. Vegans actually eat more omega-3s than meat-eaters.[28] Perhaps being a vegan makes your metabolism different. They have lower circulating levels of

---

Luan J, Wareham N, Slimani N, Rinaldi S, Couto E, Clavel-Chapelon F, Boutron-Ruault MC, Cottet V, Palli D, Agnoli C, Panico S, Tumino R, Vineis P, Agudo A, Rodriguez L, Sanchez MJ, Amiano P, Barricarte A, Huerta JM, Key TJ, Spencer EA, Bueno-de-Mesquita B, Büchner FL, Orfanos P, Naska A, Trichopoulou A, Rohrmann S, Hermann S, Boeing H, Buijsse B, Johansson I, Hellstrom V, Manjer J, Wirfält E, Jakobsen MU, Overvad K, Tjonneland A, Halkjaer J, Lund E, Braaten T, Engeset D, Odysseos A, Riboli E, Peeters PH. Meat consumption and prospective weight change in participants of the EPIC-PANACEA study. Am J Clin Nutr. 2010 Aug;92(2):398-407.

[26] Kahleova H, Hlozkova A, Fleeman R, Fletcher K, Holubkov R, Barnard ND. Fat Quantity and Quality, as Part of a Low-Fat, Vegan Diet, Are Associated with Changes in Body Composition, Insulin Resistance, and Insulin Secretion. A 16-Week Randomized Controlled Trial. Nutrients. 2019 Mar 13;11(3). pii: E615. doi: 10.3390/nu11030615.

[27] Gogga P, Śliwińska A, Aleksandrowicz-Wrona E, Małgorzewicz S. Association between different types of plant-based diets and leptin levels in healthy volunteers. Acta Biochim Pol. 2019 Feb 15;66(1):77-82.

[28] Ibid.

leptin (a hormone related to hunger and fat storage) and vegans have lower body fat.[29] These changes give vegans lower risk factors for heart disease including lower rates of high blood pressure, improper total cholesterol and LDL-cholesterol levels, BMIs, and waist circumference measurements.[30] Vegans also have lower risks of all cancers, diabetes, diverticular disease (bulges in the walls of the large intestine causing pain and other symptoms), and cataracts.[31] Their overall longevity is also longer than the general population.[32] Vegetarian diets can offer protection against "cardiovascular diseases, cardiometabolic risk factors, some cancers and total mortality," but vegan diets "offer additional protection for obesity, hypertension, type-2 diabetes, and cardiovascular mortality."[33]

It has been estimated that vegan diets can reduce the risk of coronary heart disease events (heart attack or cardiac death) by forty percent and the risk of cerebral vascular disease (stroke) by twenty nine percent.[34] Plant-based diets (the new scientific lingo for not alienating those who do not like the term vegan) also reduce the risk of metabolic syndrome and type-2 diabetes, and can reverse atherosclerosis and improve blood lipids and blood pressure.[35]

Vegan meals may also increase satiety leading to an easier time with weight loss and diabetes management. In a study of

---

[29] Ibid.

[30] Matsumoto S, Beeson WL, Shavlik DJ, Siapco G, Jaceldo-Siegl K, Fraser G, Knutsen SF. Association between vegetarian diets and cardiovascular risk factors in non-Hispanic white participants of the Adventist Health Study-2. J Nutr Sci. 2019 Feb 21;8:e6.

[31] Appleby PN, Key TJ. The long-term health of vegetarians and vegans. Proc Nutr Soc. 2016 Aug;75(3):287-93

[32] Ibid.

[33] Le LT, Sabaté J. Beyond meatless, the health effects of vegan diets: findings from the Adventist cohorts. Nutrients. 2014 May 27;6(6):2131-47.

[34] Kahleova H, Levin S, Barnard N. Cardio-Metabolic Benefits of Plant-Based Diets. Nutrients. 2017 Aug 9;9(8).

[35] Ibid.

different groups of healthy, obese, and diabetic men, satiety was greatest after consuming a vegan meal when comparing calorically and macronutrient (carbohydrate, fat, and protein) equal meals due to increases in gut hormones.[36] Vegan diets have been show to lower body weight, decrease fat mass, and improve insulin markers in a clinical trial of just sixteen weeks.[37] The authors state that deceased leucine was associated with improved BMIs and that decreased histidine was associated with decreased insulin resistance.[38] Leucine is particularly high in beef, chicken, pork, fish, cheese, and seafood. Histidine is high in beef, lamb, pork, chicken, turkey, fish, cheese, and eggs. Perhaps these foods aren't so great for us after all and are not the ones to be eating more of when we want to lose weight and be healthy long-term.

Obesity is a disease of inflammation and thus a long-term risk for other diseases. Plant-based diets have been associated with reductions in the average concentrations of C-reactive protein, interleukin-6, and soluble intercellular adhesion molecule 1. That is, they improve the inflammatory profiles of obese individuals switching to a vegan diet.[39] That is, a vegan diet can reduce systemic inflammation[40] and just may help you feel better overall. Vegans score better on the Dietary

---

[36] Klementova M, Thieme L, Haluzik M, Pavlovicova R, Hill M, Pelikanova T, Kahleova H. A Plant-Based Meal Increases Gastrointestinal Hormones and Satiety More Than an Energy- and Macronutrient-Matched Processed-Meat Meal in T2D, Obese, and Healthy Men: A Three-Group Randomized Crossover Study. Nutrients. 2019 Jan 12;11(1).

[37] Kahleova H, Fleeman R, Hlozkova A, Holubkov R, Barnard ND. A plant-based diet in overweight individuals in a 16-week randomized clinical trial: metabolic benefits of plant protein. Nutr Diabetes. 2018 Nov 2;8(1):58.

[38] Ibid.

[39] Eichelmann F, Schwingshackl L, Fedirko V, Aleksandrova K. Effect of plant-based diets on obesity-related inflammatory profiles: a systematic review and meta-analysis of intervention trials. Obes Rev. 2016 Nov;17(11):1067-1079.

[40] Sutliffe JT, Wilson LD, de Heer HD, Foster RL, Carnot MJ. C-reactive protein response to a vegan lifestyle intervention. Complement Ther Med. 2015 Feb;23(1):32-7.

Inflammatory Index (DII) which measures the association of know dietary factors which influence inflammation and may be associated with cancer. This DII measures both good and bad components of the diet and is based on peer review of over 6,500 research articles[41]. Vegans have more of the good and less of the bad, and therefore less inflammation.[42] That is, vegan food contains more anti-inflammatory factors (like phytochemicals, micronutrients, fiber, whole grains, and specific herbs and spices) and less pro-inflammatory factors (like saturated fatty acids, trans fatty acids, and cholesterol). And you can't just eat one or two things to get the effect; a vegan diet overall is likely more important than just one constituent.[43] A vegan diet could make you feel good now and for years to come.

<u>Animal Product You Should Skip.</u>
I am very sorry. I know, I just told you not to give yourself a list of things that you shouldn't do, but I'm going to do it anyway. You knew I would have to at some point. We'll talk more about all the wonderful foods you can include in your new plant-based diet, but for now, let's talk about what you should be skipping. The single biggest change you can make

---

[41] Nitin Shivappa, Susan E Steck, Thomas G Hurley, James R Hussey, and James R Hébert. Designing and developing a literature-derived, population-based dietary inflammatory index. Public Health Nutr. 2014 Aug; 17(8): 1689–1696.

[42] Ibid. The DII includes calories, carbohydrates, protein, total fat, saturated fat, alcohol, B12, B6, B-carotene, caffeine, cholesterol, fiber, folic acid, eugenol, garlic, ginger, magnesium, iron, monounsaturated fatty acids, niacin, omega-3 fatty acids, omega-6 fatty acids, polyunsaturated fatty acids, onion, selenium, saffron, thiamin, vitamins A, C, D, and E, zinc, green tea, black tea, flavan-3-ol, flavones, flavanols, flavanones, anthocyanidins, isoflavones, pepper, saffron, thyme, oregano, and rosemary.

[43] Susan Steck, PhD, MPH, RD. The Dietary Inflammatory Index: a new tool for assessing inflammatory potential of diet and associations with cancer. American Institute for Cancer Research. http://www.aicr.org/assets/docs/pdf/research/rescon2014/steck_dietary-inflammatory-index.pdf

toward a healthy weight is skipping animal products. You can skip them all together, or you can skip them any amount you like. The more you eliminate them though, the further along you will be towards your goals.

For now, let's start with a list so you can get started. You can try to avoid or eliminate these animal products in any order you wish. Most people start with the elimination of red meats or all meat products. The choice is up to you. The more that product has been contributing to excess calories, and food cravings, the greater the elimination of that food should make toward your weight loss goals. Later, I'll go into more specifics as to why these items should be avoided.

Given our current state of knowledge, the foods that are the major contributors to excess calories, fats, and toxins are the following which should be avoided as much as possible. Please start the process now of avoiding as many of these overweight and obesity related foods as possible:

- Meats and Meat fats: This includes beef, ham, lamb, pork, veal, game including bison, rabbit, venison, luncheon and deli meats, lard, tallow, gelatin, sausage, frankfurters, hotdogs, liver and other organ meat, and other forms of meat.

- Poultry: This includes chicken, duck, goose, turkey, quail, ground chicken and turkey, and any other bird in whatever form.

- Fish: This includes fish, like catfish, cod, flounder, haddock, halibut, herring, mackerel, pollock, porgy, salmon, bass, snapper, swordfish, trout, tuna, canned fish like anchovies, clams, tuna, sardines, as well as shellfish, such as clams, crab, crayfish, lobster, mussels, octopus, oysters, scallops, squid (calamari), shrimp, caviar, and other ocean creatures.

- Milk and other Dairy Products: This includes all dairy, including milk, cream, sour cream, crème fraiche, buttermilk, milk powder (or powdered milk), milk containing protein powders, condensed milk, evaporated milk, butter, ghee, clarified butter, milk fat, cheese, whey, casein (caseinates, milk protein concentrates and isolates, whey protein concentrates and isolates, hydrolysates, mineral concentrates), cottage cheese, cream cheese, yogurt, lassi, gelato, ice cream, ice milk, frozen custard, frozen yogurt, and other cheeses and products made from cow's milk or any other kind of milk.

- Eggs: This includes chicken eggs, duck eggs, Egg Beaters, reduced cholesterol eggs, and all types of eggs, whether prepared on their own or included in a recipe.

- Fried Foods: Including French fries, onion rings, potato chips, corn chips, other chips, cheese puffs or cheese curls, fried pork rinds, doughnuts, fried mozzarella sticks, fried zucchini, tempura, fried rice, potato skins, fried dough, funnel cakes, fried fish, fish and chips, fried bananas or plantains, chicken fried steak, chicken wings, corn dogs, fried calamari, fried chicken, fried shrimp, clams, scallops, or oysters, hushpuppies, hash browns, fried ice cream, fried mushrooms, Scotch eggs, fried turkey, or other fried foods.

In fact, the single most food linked to obesity is chips.[44] So,

---

[44] Dariush Mozaffarian, M.D., Dr. P.H., Tao Hao, M.P.H., Eric B. Rimm, Sc.D., Walter C. Willett, M.D., Dr.P.H., and Frank B. Hu, M.D., Ph.D. Changes in Diet and Lifestyle and Long-Term Weight Gain in Women and Men. June 23, 2011, N Engl J Med 2011; 364:2392-2404.

please avoid chips! It doesn't help that the food industry keeps adding all kinds of new flavors of chips either. This is called line-extension and this practice has grown extensively in recent years as food scientists keep creating new ways of artificially producing flavors of natural foods cheaply. The growth of potato chip sales is linked to both the demand for quick snacks and increasing flavor varieties. In fact, while potato chip sales have gone up at a rate of 4.4 percent, flavored variety sales have increased at a rate of 5.8 percent per year.[45] No wonder we are getting fatter as a nation.

Other forms of potatoes rank up there in other foods making people fat, too, but you bet people aren't eating them as plain potatoes. Other foods highly associated with weight gain include "sugar-sweetened beverages, unprocessed red meats, and processed meats," plus lifestyle factors of alcohol use, more than eight hours or less than six hours of sleep per night, television watching, and smoking.[46] The consumption of vegetables, whole grains, fruit, and nuts are negatively associated with weight gain, as are physical activity and sleeping between six and eight hours per night.[47]

<u>Nutrient Poor, White Foods That You Should Skip.</u>
You should also try to skip anything that is made with anything white or heavily refined. Not only is this because I am a nutritionist, and I want you to eat the healthiest foods, but because these foods tend to be loaded with extra calories that you don't need, chemicals that stimulate your appetite and taste perception, and tend to contain many of the animal products listed above. Eliminating these foods will eliminate a lot of junk. While I do agree that you should skip the foods that we

---

[45] U.S. Potato Chips Market To See 4.4% Sales Gains By 2025. Data & Insights. Candy & Snack Today, October 31, 2018.
[46] Dariush Mozaffarian, M.D., Dr.P.H., Tao Hao, M.P.H., Eric B. Rimm, Sc.D., Walter C. Willett, M.D., Dr.P.H., and Frank B. Hu, M.D., Ph.D. Changes in Diet and Lifestyle and Long-Term Weight Gain in Women and Men. June 23, 2011, N Engl J Med 2011; 364:2392-2404.
[47] Ibid.

have mentioned already above first, especially the meats, the next step and logical progression of becoming healthier is to kick out everything that is processed white. That is:

- White flour: Including items marked white flour, flour, wheat flour, bread flour, cake flour, all-purpose flour, plain flour, bromated flour, unbleached flour, pastry flour, cookie flour, cracker flour, self-rising or raising flour, durum flour, high gluten flour, and other white flours,

- White pasta: Including any shape or size made from white flour, durum wheat, gnocchi made from white potatoes and flour, rice pasta, ramen, or soba,

- White rice: Including parboiled rice, polished rice, rice flour, rice noodles, white Basmati, Thai rice, sticky rice, puffed white rice, and other white rice products,

- White sugar: Including table sugar, sucrose, beet sugar, palm sugar, sugar cane, brown sugar, corn syrup, high fructose corn syrup, evaporated cane sugar, dextrose, confectionary sugar, 10x sugar, raw sugar, turbinado sugar, cane juice, demerara, muscovado, mill white sugar, plantation sugar, crystal sugar, superior sugar, white refined sugar, granulated sugar, powdered sugar, rock candy, sugar syrup, pancake syrup, or products made from these sugars whether they are organic or not,

- And anything made from these foods, including bread, cakes, crackers, pastries, brownies, bars, puddings, etc.

Now don't get discouraged. I know it seems like a lot. But as you become healthier and more particular in your food choices, these will become foods that you will not want to eat anyway, or items that you only eat on occasion.

Let's look at some examples of why you should skip these.

<u>Why Meat Does Not Belong on Your Slimming Plan.</u>

First off, results don't lie. Everyone who responded to my study lost weight when they stopped eating meats. The more they ate, the more they lost when they eliminated it. The less of them they ate, the more weight they took off. The longer they stayed away from eating it, the longer they kept the weight off.

Now there are lots of different types of meat, and I am sure that you have heard why you should eat them, for you iron, or your energy, or because your ancestors did, or whatever. Let's take a skeptical look.

Let's start by looking at ground beef. Ground beef is classified into three types: regular which is 27 percent fat, lean which is 21 percent fat, and extra lean which is 17 percent fat. A serving is considered three (3) ounces, which by most people's standards would be on the small side. If you took each of these and broiled them medium, the regular fat would be 17.6 grams of fat or 65percent of calories from fat. The lean would be 15.7 grams of fat or 61 percent of calories from fat. The extra lean would be 13.9 grams of fat or 58 percent of calories from fat. No matter how you cut it, beef is not a low-fat or low-calorie food. You may cut 3.7 grams of fat by going from the regular to the extra lean, but 58 percent of calories from fat does not constitute a low-fat food. The government defines low fat as "not more than 30 percent of calories from fat."[48] In my opinion, even that is very high. Over half of calories from fat does not cut it. If you're eating out, don't bet on getting the extra lean either. Most people like the taste of fat, so restaurants are not going to use the extra lean if they are most concerned with taste. In fact, gourmet steak, and even burgers these days, are cooked with extra fat and even a dollop of butter on top! And what about the calories? Remember, there are nine (9) calories per gram of fat, so you are getting 158.4 calories, 141.3 calories, and 125.1 calories from fat for

---

[48] http://www.cfsan.fda.gov/~dms/flg-6a.html, U.S. Food and Drug Administration, Center for Food Safety and Applied Nutrition, A Food Labeling Guide, September 1994.

each of these respectively. And remember, that is in just three ounces. Most burgers are six ounces, so all those numbers would be double!

Now let's look at something that everyone thinks vegetarians eat a lot of: Tofu. Tofu comes in different varieties also. Tofu can be high fat, too. Let's look at two varieties: Regular and Light. Let's use the same size serving, 3 ounces. The regular tofu contains 53 percent fat, again not exactly a low-fat food. However, this translates to only 5.9 grams of fat or 53.1 calories. The Light variety is 24 percent fat. This is only one (1) gram of fat or 9 calories. The tofu also has only 0.9 grams and 0.7 grams of saturated fat respectively. The beef contains 6.9 grams, 6.2 grams, and 5.5 grams of saturated fat respectively. Saturated fat is that most responsible for elevating blood cholesterol (LDL) and the greatest dietary predictor of cardiovascular (heart) disease. So naturally, if you must choose between the ground beef and the tofu, you would want to choose the tofu – but what about the taste? Let's work on that by showing you a more reasonable comparison than just plain ground beef verses just plain tofu.

Let's use chili as an example. Regular beef-based chili with beans contains 59 percent fat or 26 grams fat (234 calories). Tofu chili contains 22 percent fat or 6 grams fat (54 calories). You save 180 calories by skipping the meat. If you like chili, take your tofu from the package, rinse it off, smush the whole thing with your hand into crumbles, and use it instead of meat in your chili. My mom always said that she liked tofu hot dogs because she couldn't tell the difference between them and "the real thing" after you put the ketchup, mustard, and whatever else on them. It's the same thing with the chili, there so many spices and beans in the chili that you won't miss the meat.

What about low-fat meats? The trend in the general public has been towards lower fat foods, yes, but are they really low-fat? Everyone for some reason wants to hold on to the meat. We have looked at one example above, with ground beef, about why even "extra lean" doesn't mean low fat. What about if we trade one kind of meat for another?

They call pork: "The other white meat." So, let's look at pork. A pork chop is 54 percent fat and 10 grams fat if you eat just three ounces. A pork chop is considered to be 6 ounces though, so you are eating 20 grams of fat or 180 calories just from fat, and 8 of those grams are from saturated fat. Braised pork loin is 72 percent fat and 21.6 grams of fat (or 194.4 calories) in just a 3-ounce serving. 8.1 grams of this are saturated fat. Roasted pork ribs are 21.5 grams of fat (7.8 grams of which are saturated fat) and a whopping 71 percent of calories from fat. Doesn't sound like pork is so low in fat.

Let's look at chicken. If you average out all of the parts and roast it, a "roaster" chicken would be 56 percent fat or 11.4 of fat in three ounces (102.6 calories including 3 grams of saturated fat), and a "stewing"[49] chicken would be 61 percent fat or 16 grams of fat in three ounces (144 calories including 4.3 grams of saturated fat). This does not include any of the sauces or deep frying or breading or anything that so many people like.

Now let look at what everybody lately thinks is just so healthy: fish. Don't make it breaded or fried or any of those fat adding ways of cooking that people like. Let's take a plain three-ounce piece of baked salmon. It happens to be 54 percent fat with 10.5 grams of fat or 94.5 calories from fat including 2.1 grams of saturated fat – not so great in just a three-ounce piece. Eating out you might get double that.

<u>Why Milk and Eggs Don't Belong Either.</u>
So, what about milk? When you read on the label that you are buying 1 percent or 2 percent milk, most people think you are buying a low-fat food. Don't be fooled though! One percent and two percent are the percentage of milk by volume that is fat, not the percentage of calories that are fat. Let's start with whole milk. Whole milk has about 50 percent of its calories from fat, with about 157 calories in a cup of milk. So

---

[49] This is what the nutrition reference books and the food industry call them. This is not my terminology and I find it an awful way to refer to an animal.

called "low-fat 2% milk" contains 34 percent of calories from fat with 121 calories in a cup of milk. So called "low-fat 1% milk" contains 22 percent of calories from fat with 102 calories per cup of milk. Even "skim or nonfat" milk, which you would think has no fat in it, contains 5 percent of calories from fat with 86 calories in a cup.

Let's now look at eggs. A whole chicken egg is 86 calories with 61 percent fat. Few people eat only one egg at a sitting though and few people have eggs without making them into something else first. If you do anything but boil or poach them, you are likely to add oil or butter in the cooking process, or something else like cheese or bacon bits as a filling; either way you are adding fat. Egg whites contain less than one percent fat, but to most people they are not very palatable.

Why Skip the Fried Foods?

When it comes to fried foods, frying can make just about anything taste good from dough to an old boot. Frying obviously adds fat. Fat adds calories, but it also creates toxins known as advanced glycogen end products (AGEs) or glycotoxins. These toxins accumulate in the body and create oxidative stress causing cell damage. This oxidative stress has been associated with many diseases including diabetes and cardiovascular disease,[50] inflammatory responses, oxidative stress, and aging.[51]

Examine What You Eat Now.

Try this exercise. This is what we call a 24-hour food recall. If you have started taking photos of everything you have

---

[50] http://www.insidermedicine.ca/daily-health-videos, "BBQ Foods Potentially Linked to Aging and Diabetes ", Dr. Joanna Oliver, April 27, 2007

[51] Circulating glycotoxins and dietary advanced glycation end products: two links to inflammatory response, oxidative stress, and aging. J Gerontol A Biol Sci Med Sci. 2007 Apr;62(4):427-33. PMID: 17452738 [PubMed - indexed for MEDLINE]. Uribarri J, Cai W, Peppa M, Goodman S, Ferrucci L, Striker G, Vlassara H.

been eating, this exercise will be easy. Just look at the photos you took, or if not, just record as you go through the day. Since it is sometimes hard to remember exactly what you are the day before and we tend to underestimate, record as you go rather than trying to remember. Be honest with yourself.

Write down everything you ate and the amount you ate for the last 24 hours. Try and be as accurate as you can. Don't try and change things based on what you just read or if you are feeling guilty. Include everything. Did you have drinks or snacks in between meals? Did you add sugar of cream to your coffee? Did you put butter or jelly on your toast? Try to remember the first thing you had to eat when you woke up and think through the day about what you did and where you were to help you remember what you ate. If you normally eat three meals a day, try to include all three meals in your 24-hour recall. That is, if you haven't eaten lunch yet today, be sure to include what you ate yesterday for lunch. Include a whole 24 hours and don't worry if it was a typical day or not. Just write down everything you ate. Also, if you haven't made any of the changes to your diet we have just talked about, that is fine. Don't feel guilty. Be honest and use this exercise as a learning tool to help you see what you have currently been consuming. For now, fill in the columns labeled "Food I Ate" and "How Much I Ate." We'll talk about the last column later. (Another copy of this appears in the Appendix.)

24-Hour Food Recall

Food Eaten	Amount	This Counts As

Now think about these foods and how you feel about them? Was there anything going on that made you want to eat them or eat too much? Were you bored? Were you upset? Should you be eating them? How did they make you feel? Did you feel good after you ate them? Did you want to take a nap after you ate or were you full of energy? Did you eat too much? What might you differently?

<u>Categorizing Your Diet</u>
Just for starters, a basic way of looking at our diets is by using the Food Guide Pyramid as developed by the U.S. Department of Agriculture and the U.S. Department of Health and Human Services. The Pyramid uses basic categories to determine approximate ranges of appropriate intake for calories and nutrient consumption. By looking at you diet in comparison to the Pyramid, you can get a basic idea of where to start with making changes to your diet.

This Pyramid has change over time. In fact, it wasn't a pyramid at fit at all. It was a circle, called "The Basic Seven," and looked like this:

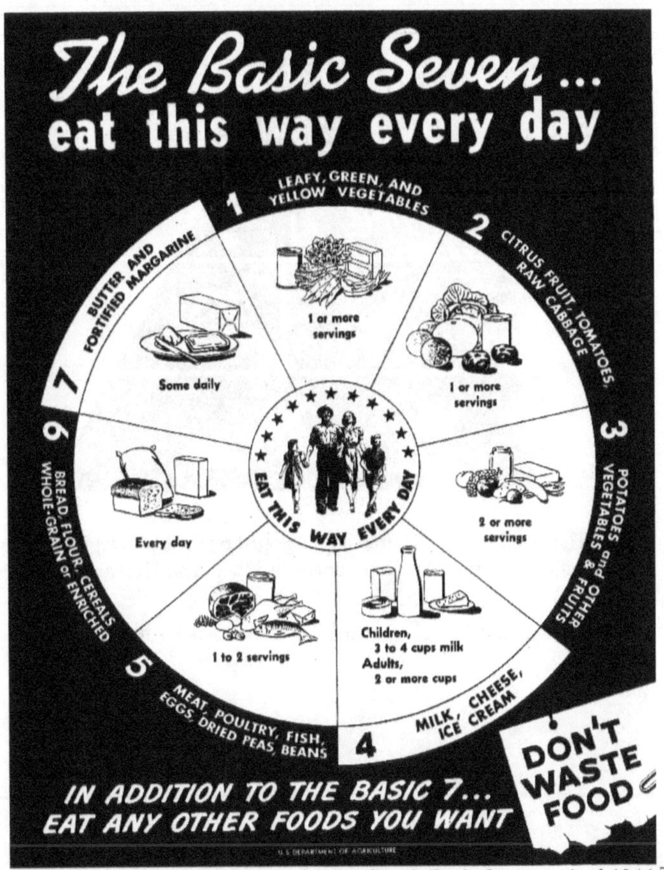

The United States Department of Agriculture's Basic Seven revised 1946.[52]

A later incarnation was the "Food Guide Pyramid," which looked like this:

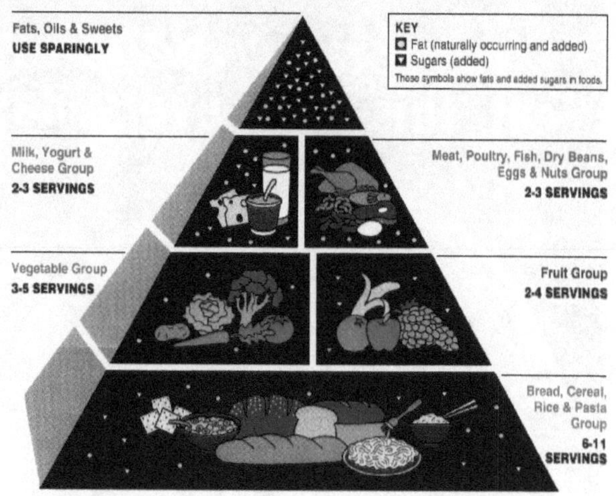

The Food Guide Pyramid as developed by the U.S. Department of Agriculture and the U.S. Department of Health and Human Services.[53]

Then we had "MyPyramid," which looked like this:

---

[53] Public domain. https://upload.wikimedia.org/wikipedia/commons/6/6d/USDA_Food_Pyramid.gif

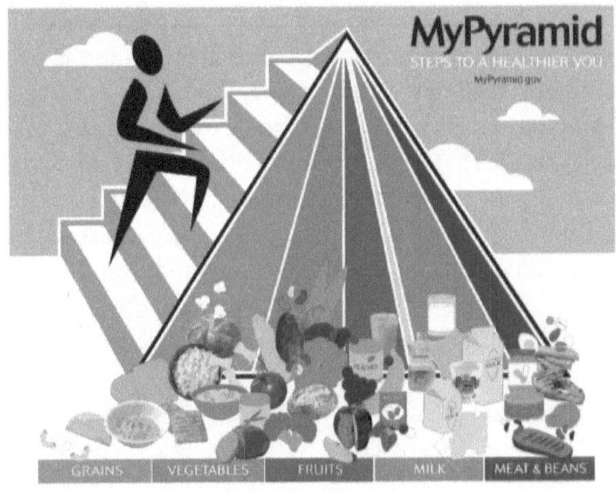

Food Guide Pyramid, Center for Nutrition Policy and Promotion, USDA[54]

And now there's "MyPlate," which looks like this:

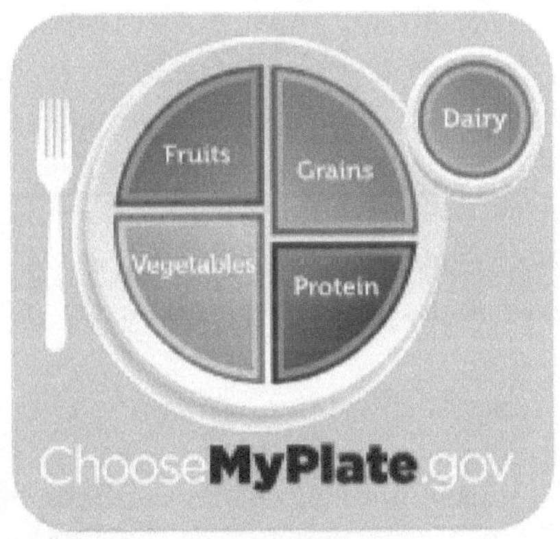

USDA's MyPlate.[55]

---

[54] Public Domain/USDA.
https://commons.wikimedia.org/wiki/File:MyPyramidFood.svg
[55] Public Domain/USDA.
https://commons.wikimedia.org/wiki/File:USDA_MyPlate_green.svg

Now, before we look at how you ate compares to these, let's look at the evolution of the graphics and the food that our government feels we should have. The first thing I notice is that they have really been dumbed down over the years. They seem to think that fewer words should be used with simpler graphics. In fact, the main graphics have eliminated numbers altogether. (You can, if you look elsewhere, find recommendations on serving sizes and servings per day though.) You also see poor grammar. As far as I am concerned, running words together isn't acceptable. Anyway, let's compare what we can.

Can you believe that the first food the government wanted us to have in 1946 was leafy, green, and yellow vegetables! That's right. They were listed number one. They wanted us to have:

- One or more servings of leafy, green, and yellow vegetables,
- One or more servings of citrus fruit, tomatoes, or raw cabbage,
- Two or more servings of potatoes and other vegetables or fruits,
- Two or more cups of milk, cream, or ice cream (for adults),
- One or two servings of meat, poultry, fish, eggs, dried peas, or beans,
- Bread, flour, or cereals, whole-grain or enriched every day,
- And some daily butter or fortified margarine.

It is really amazing the emphasis the Basic Seven placed on vegetables. Then things switched to the Food Guide Pyramid with:

- Six to eleven servings of bread, cereal, rice, or pasta,
- Three to five servings of vegetables,
- Two to four servings of fruit,
- Two to three servings of milk, yogurt, or cheese,

- Two to three servings of meat, poultry, fish, dry beans, eggs, or nuts,
- And fats, oils, and sweets sparingly.

Now the first thing you likely notice is that grains are at the bottom and animal products are at the top. Perhaps this showed their superiority and gave built-in bias. It also was criticized for having grains as its base and blamed for making America fat along with the low-fat craze along with sugar. We never were low-fat though and the low-fat commercial products we consumed as a nation were loaded with sugar "to make up for missing the taste of the fat." Please note most of the food industry thinks that things don't taste good unless they have salt, sugar, and fat. Quite a mixed message though saying to use fat sparingly, yet putting it at the top, the pinnacle of the pyramid.

The first thing I notice between the Basic Seven and the Food Guide Pyramid is how much the serving size went up. They didn't used to tell you how many breads and cereals to eat, then they started to tell us six to eleven. The number of dairy servings went up, as did the number of protein servings. Notice too, that the type of fruit and vegetable used to be specified, and then it wasn't anymore. Sweets weren't even mentioned on the Basic Seven, and butter and margarine were mentioned so that vitamin A was included for sure. Now, of course, we don't mention margarine anymore, because we all know that margarine contains trans-fatty acids which increase the incidence of heart disease. Perhaps the government should not have told us just how many servings to eat, however, since most of our weights went up during this time.

Let look at the MyPyramid now. We kept the pyramid shape but notice now that serving size is no longer included on the basic graphic. The pyramid has also been turned on its side. Perhaps they though one food group should not be the base of the diet, or one food group should not be deemed as superior due to its positioning at the top of the pyramid. We are supposed to notice the size difference between the different food groups and somehow register this into our daily food consumption. All rather confusing if you ask me. One major difference too, that a big deal was made of at the time was the incorporation of activity into the graphic. Too bad it never said just how much activity we should get nor how many serving we should get of certain foods.[56] Perhaps people felt that if you ate this way you should feel like being more active.

Lastly, we have MyPlate. Here our serving plate is divided so that we can see how much of our plate each meal should be of each food group. I don't know about you, but I certainly don't eat this way. Very rarely will I have all these things on my plate at once, much less accompanied by a dairy-type side or drink. This way of serving requires a lot of prep-work on the part of the cook, and the only time you can be sure that I eat this way is at big holidays and family gatherings. If I cooked this way all of the time, I would have leftovers in my refrigerator all of the time and I would wind-up being the only one that would eat them, because I don't know about your family, but my family would rather help themselves to something else than eat leftovers for even one night.

So MyPlate attempts to show us that most of the foods we eat should be fruits and vegetable, but it fails to tell us what types. Indeed, this is what all these food guides have attempted to tell us. The Basic Seven in my estimation does so the best job. We want to make sure that the diet of the population includes all the nutrients needed to meet basic daily requirements for all the nutrients to prevent deficiency and meet energy requirements. I say population because these are not meant to meet the requirement of every individual. There could be either deficiencies (unlikely) or excesses (quite possibly). With this in mind, each food group is devised and recommended. Meat for protein. Dairy for calcium. Fruit for vitamins, especially vitamin C. Vegetable for fiber and vitamins, especially folic acid. Grains for energy and fiber.

---

[56] This is of course in the main graphic. They did say these things elsewhere in their recommendations, but you had to look for them.

Now, you could divide foods up into all different groups. The food groups that the government uses and promotes are influenced by all sorts of factors (e.g. lobbying, current research, popular opinion, etc.). This does not mean that this is how we should do it now or will do it in the future. Perhaps, we could divide the diet into cancer promotors and inhibitors, or nutrient dense foods and nutrient poor foods, or filling foods and foods that make you want to eat more (obesogens).

I used to work for the WIC Program. This is the United Stated Department of Agriculture's (USDA) Special Supplemental Food Program for Women, Infants, and Children (WIC). It works to ensure the nutritional adequacy of pregnant and lactating low-income women, their infants, and children less than five years old. The program monitors growth and nutritional adequacy to prevent health problems in the populations they serve, while at the same time promoting the foods that the USDA promotes. How WIC looks at the nutritional adequacy of these populations is still to me the best way to look at the quality of the diet.

Foods are in the WIC program according the necessary nutrients they supply in the diet and assessment is done according to which of these foods participants eat. WIC asks specifically for foods that supply protein, calcium, vitamin A (or beta carotene), folic acid, iron, fiber, and calories. The total quantity of calories and the intake of empty calories are assessed.

You can do something like this with your 24-hour recall you did above. Go back and categorize what you ate according to the follow important foods. That is, give them a reason for being there according to the nutrients they supply, or if they do not supply anything of value. I know all of these foods aren't vegan yet, but I am assuming you aren't yet either. Just play along and mark them as:

- Foods High in Protein: Meats, beans, nuts, legumes, soy.
- Foods High in Calcium: Dairy, tofu, leafy green vegetables, whole grains.

- Foods High in Vitamin A or Beta-Carotene: Yellow and orange vegetables including squash, sweet potatoes.
- Foods High in Folic Acid: Leafy green vegetables, whole grains.
- Foods High in Iron: Meats, beans, legumes.
- Foods High in Fiber: Whole fruits, vegetables, and whole grains, nuts.
- Foods High in Calories and not much else: Fried foods, white baked goods, sweets, and candy.

Go back now and see what you ate and approximately how they fit into these groups. As you well know, just because a food fits into one of these groups does not mean it does not fit into one of the others as well. Do your best.

Another way to categorize you diet might be this:

- Real Food: Anything produced by nature.
- Junk Food: Anything with mostly processed ingredients, fat, sugar, or man-made substances.

Go back now and see what happens. And what do you think?

You could also try grouping what you eat according to the government's recommendations. Next to what you ate fill in first how what group the food you ate counts as. You can pretty much count things using common sense, meat in meat/proteins, bread in grains, etc. But if they happen to be laden with fat, oil, or sugar, count them as a fat, oil, or sweet. For example, if you had pork rinds don't count them as a meat group, count them as a fat. If you had a donut or pastry, don't count it as a bread, cereal, rice, or pasta group, count it as a sweet. If you had fruit chews, fruit leather, or a fruit drink with hardly any fruit in it at all, don't count it as a fruit group, count it as a fat, oil, or sweet.

Now that you have figured out which category the foods you ate fall into, in several different ways, let's figure out how many servings of each you had. Use this basic guideline to write down the number of servings you ate next on your chart:

For the Bread, Grain, Cereal and Pasta Group,
- 1 slice of bread,
- 1/2 cup of rice, cooked cereal or pasta,
- 1 cup of ready-to-eat cereal, or
- 1 tortilla count as one serving.

For Fruits and Vegetables:
- 1 cup of raw leafy vegetables,
- 1/2 cup of other vegetables, cooked or raw,
- 3/4 cup of vegetable juice,
- one medium apple, orange, or banana,
- 1/2 cup of chopped, cooked or canned fruit, or
- 3/4 cup of fruit juice count as one serving.

For Meat, Poultry, Fish, Dry Beans, Eggs, and Nuts, the following count as a serving:
- 2-3 ounces of cooked lean meat, poultry, or fish,
- One egg,
- 2 tablespoons of peanut butter,
- 1/2 cup cooked dry beans,
- 1/3 cup of nuts.

For Milk, Yogurt, and Cheese,
- 1 cup of milk or yogurt,
- 1 1/2 ounces of natural cheese,
- 2 ounces of process cheese count as a serving.

<u>How Does What You Eat Compare?</u>
Just how does what you eat compare to what is recommended? Well, if you are like most people who want to lose weight, and most Americans in fact, most of what you ate came from meats, dairy, processed baked goods, and sweets. Most Americans eat few if any fruits and vegetables, and most

of those we eat are processed potatoes and fruit juices, especially orange juice. We eat more servings than necessary of most everything except the things we should. If we really look at the serving sizes listed above, we eat even more than we think.

If you want to do this again to compare other days and what you ate, go right ahead. The more days you do this for, the better idea you will get about just what you are eating on a regular basis and where you can make improvements.

Why Not Just Go by the Government's Food Guide Pyramid?

What a question! First off, the pyramid is not intended for weight loss. And second, and even more importantly, the pyramid is full of political compromises. In 1991, I was at an event at a major university in Boston while getting my Master of Science in Nutrition. All these big shots in the nutrition research were there and the speaker was saying that in order to have the lowest risk of disease the government's recommendation for fat intake should be only ten percent of the diet. This provoked some discussion. Americans ate on average about forty percent fat at the time,[57] and some were eating about fifty percent. What was amazing to me was that they all agreed that the recommendation should be 10 percent of calories from fat! I couldn't believe it. I was stunned. How could it be then that the research said one thing and the government recommended another? They went on to agree that since Americans were eating so much fat and that the discrepancy between how much people were eating and what the best recommendation would be was so great, that they could never make such a recommendation since Americans would never believe another thing they said, much less what

---

[57] As of the NHANES 1999-2000 study, Americans were eating thirty three percent fat.
National Health and Nutrition Examination Survey. Intake of Calories and Selected Nutrients for the United States Population, 1999-2000. https://www.cdc.gov/nchs/data/nhanes/databriefs/calories.pdf

would the meat, dairy, and fast food industries have to say about it!

So, if you've been reading all those diet books that say that we as Americans all gained weight on a "low-fat diet" and now we should be eating protein, they are all wrong! Americans have never been on a low-fat diet! "Low-fat" was used as a marketing tool to push convenience foods. With very few exceptions, low-fat meant that processed sugar was added in its place. Salt was added, too. The food industry, again with little exception, thinks that the only things that sell are salt, sugar, and fat. No wonder weights stayed the same or went up. We ate more and more sugar, more and more processed foods, few and fewer fruits and vegetables, more and more sodium, and less and less fiber, all while never being low-fat. The food industry thinks that salt, sugar, and fat sell. And they do, because to most people they taste good. But what they are learning more and more is that healthy, low-fat, low-salt, low-fat foods taste good, too. And they taste much better when you eat them all the time.

Not only can you lose weight by making the change to a diet low in animal products, but you can dramatically change your overall health, your risk for serious disease, and increase your energy level. By becoming a vegetarian and then progressing to a vegan, you can dramatically cut your intake of unhealthy fats, excess calories, and lose weight, all while increasing your intake of the healthy, lifegiving substances that have been shown to decrease your risk of chronic disease, including diabetes, heart disease, and cancer.

So, let's look at your intake from your 24-hour food record one more time. Ask yourself the following questions to see just how nutritious your current diet is.

Are you eating:

- Something with vitamin C daily? This could be fruit (such as citrus, kiwis, papaya, cantaloupe, strawberries, etc.) or vegetable (such as bell pepper, broccoli, kale, cauliflower, Brussel sprouts, chili peppers, etc.)

- Something high in iron? (soybeans, tofu, beans, chickpeas, lentils, whole grains, sunflower seeds, nuts, sesame seeds, tahini, cashews, almonds, leafy greens, prune juice, etc.)
- Something high in protein? (beans, nuts, soy, lentils, etc.)
- Something with omega-3 fatty acids? (flax, chia, hemp, leafy greens, algae, walnuts, soy, beans,
- Something high in vitamin A? (carrots, sweet potato, cantaloupe, apricots, kale, spinach, romaine lettuce, peppers, etc.)
- Lots of things with fiber? (whole grains, fruit, vegetables, nuts, seeds, legumes, beans, etc.)
- Foods high in phytonutrients? (Plants nutrients associated with color including those in kale, blueberries, pomegranate, fruits, vegetables, nuts, beans, seeds, legumes, algae, and other superfoods.)

Or did you eat:
- Foods with ingredients that you can't pronounce?
- Highly processed foods?
- Deep fried foods?
- Red meat, chicken, pork, or other meats?
- Lots of dairy?
- Eggs?

Could it be that you are starving yourself for nutrients all the while you are consuming excess calories? If you are not getting a source of all the items above, your body could be telling you that it is craving more food because it is lacking in something.

Growing-up we had donkeys. My mom saved farm animals the same way other people save dogs and cats. (We had twelve dogs and almost thirty cats at one point, all with names and a story of how they were saved, too. And of course, we lived on a farm.) A man bought ten pregnant donkeys at auction and saved them from the slaughterhouse where they were headed. My mom took one and my aunt took one, too, so we both had baby donkeys born on the farm. Well, baby donkeys are the cutest thing and my little brother and I had our picture in the newspaper that year with baby Gray Cloud.

Well, donkeys also are super smart. We had barn doors with sliding locks and one-time Grey Cloud opened the barn door, let Tex (the horse) in the stall and closed the door behind him. She also used to let her mother, Dinah, in the barn to steal the grain. Well, not only did we have to put hooks on the inside of the doors, but then we had to change them out, too, because she figured them out. The only thing that stopped her was putting catches on the inside of the doors that she couldn't do without a thumb. All this being said, donkeys can chew. Our third donkey came from Death Valley. They Spaniard settlers left them there the same way they left them in the Grand Canyon. Of course, these animals were in terrible condition and after they were airlifted out of the Grand Canyon, they were airlifted out of Death Valley, too. They survived in Death Valley by chewing on wood. All the donkeys used to chew the wood around the barn, too. The fence, the doors, and the walls if they could reach them, especially in the winter. All this despite getting hay and grain. Mom also got them a salt lick. But it didn't stop until she got them a salt lick with minerals in it. By George, they knew they needed something else, and kept eating other things until they got it!

You know what, research shows humans do the same kind of thing! Humans exhibiting pica (eating nonfood substances such as dirt or chalk) often have low iron, zinc, or calcium levels and supplementation can stop the behavior.[58] Indeed,

---

[58] Nchito, Mbiko, et al. "Effects of Iron and Multimicronutrient Supplementation on Geophagy: a Two-by-Two Factorial Study among Zambian Schoolchildren in Lusaka." *Transactions of the Royal Society of Tropical Medicine and Hygiene*, vol. 98, no. 4, 2004, pp. 218–227., doi:10.1016/s0035-9203(03)00045-2.
Rabel, Antoinette, et al. "Ask about Ice, Then Consider Iron." *Journal of the American Association of Nurse Practitioners*, vol. 28, no. 2, 2016, pp.

sailors with scurvy were said to have an unnatural craving for lemons, and therefore vitamin C. Indeed, scurvy was treated with what they called "scorbutick beer" which was a combination of various seagrasses that has since been found to contain measurable amounts of vitamin C.[59] Could humans have found "scurvy grass" (*Cochlearia officinalis*, one of the ingredients in that anti-scurvy beer, related to cabbage) if not for such a craving? I don't know, but we seem to have an inborn sense about what our bodies need.

When I was in college, I was in a basic nutrition course. The professor was describing lots of different nutrients and in this discussion. She was saying that foods have a lot of other chemicals in them that have no known function. The nutrient that she named as an example was a "coloring component" and had no known function. This stuck out to me like a sore thumb. That nutrient was lycopene! Yes, lycopene has a coloring function, but today we know it is also is one of the most highly researched phytochemicals known to prevent cancer! Phytochemicals come from plants. "Phyto" means plants. These are chemicals that are in plants and many of them may be the key to both cancer prevention and treatment. Indeed, vegetarians have lower cancer rates.

There are in fact so many nutrients that science is saying are needed for the prevention of cancer and other illnesses that it would be very difficult to eat any large portion of junk and be healthy because those healthy substances come from natural plants, not anything man-made. And forget about saying, "Well, I take my vitamins." That isn't going to cut it. The nutrients work in harmony with each other and science, like my nutrition professor, may never know all the things that we

---

116–120., doi:10.1002/2327-6924.12268.

Reynolds, Ralph D. "Pagophagia and Iron Deficiency Anemia." *Annals of Internal Medicine*, vol. 69, no. 3, Jan. 1968, p. 435., doi:10.7326/0003-4819-69-3-435.

[59] Hughes, R.Elwyn. The Rise and Fall of the "Antiscorbutics": Some notes of the traditional cures for "Land Scurvy," Medical History, 1990, 34: 52-64.

do indeed need.

<u>What Should I Eat?</u>

So now that you know it can be done, what can you eat? Well let me tell you this first, one of the keys to having fun with this is how you think about things. Wait a minute – fun you say? Yes, fun! If you're not enjoying yourself and doing something you like to do, how can you stick with anything? I know if I like something, it is a whole lot easier to do something than if I think of it as drudgery. So, think of it this way: Vegetarianism means trying an abundance of new foods, not giving some up. This is something that you are going to do for yourself, not a punishment. You want to be a healthier, happier, new you.

So, what I would like to do in the coming pages is tell you about some exciting foods and ways to try them, while at the same time telling you about all of the essential nutrients that will keep you healthy and satisfied while you lose weight. For most, the radical change of eliminating animal products opens up a whole new world of ingredients.

<u>High Nutrient Foods.</u>

Eating high nutrient foods is really the key to being satisfied and not wanting to gorge on things that you really know you shouldn't. Someone asked me, "I always eat dessert because I'm still hungry. What should I do?" Well, the simple answer to that is, if your dinner is healthy, "Eat more of your dinner." That is the easy answer, but things are a little more complicated than that. For most, no matter what they have for dinner, they feel the need to have even a little bit of sweet dessert afterwards. We have something called taste satiety. That is, we get sick of eating the same thing. My ten-year old says, "I'm full," but then says she wants dessert. What she really means is, "I'm sick of eating the dinner. Give me a different taste for dessert." You can use this fact to lose weight, provided you have the willpower to eat a very limited number of foods. In fact, pretty much any food that you eat, and eat only that food exclusively for some time, will make you lose weight, just because you get sick of it. Now, I don't mean a broad category like cakes or pies. There is too much variety there, and I know I personally would never get sick of that. What I mean though are things like the ketogenic diet. You start feeling sick, and sick of it, after a while. The head of the Potato Board went on a diet of exclusively potatoes when the USDA was going to eliminate potatoes from the list of acceptable WIC foods that could be purchased. And you know what? He lost weight. Yes, a diet of exclusively potatoes can make you lose weight. And just like eating any diet that does not include variety, you probably will wind-up being nutrient deficient in something sooner or later. In fact, there is a good possibility you are nutrient deficient now and don't even know it.

Therefore, in order to be a good example of a healthy, happy plant eater, you need to learn about where specific nutrients come from. This is so that you can reap all the benefits of being a vegetarian and eventual vegan without any of the drawbacks.

Why do you have to learn this now? Well, we all learned in school where various nutrients come from. The problem was we got a biased viewpoint, and I'm going to give you a biased viewpoint now, too. The difference is that science is pointing more and more to the benefits of a plant-based diet. Notice that they are saying "plant-based." I just think that this is because they think it is a lot easier to chew, politically, than saying to stop eating animal products altogether.

The other answer to our question above about wanting to eat dessert is to include as many of the tastes in your meal as possible so that you won't be craving that sweet taste for dessert because it wasn't included in your savory dinner. If you try to include a little sweet, salt, fat, sour, bitter, and umami (savory) in your meal, you will be including all the tastes and won't be craving any other tastes for dessert.

The other thing that will help you crave less is eating more foods high in nutrients, not just calories, salt, sugar, and fat. Nutritionists talk about nutrient density. That is, how packed with nutrients a certain food is compared to how many calories it has. If you eat something that has lots of calories, but comparably few nutrients, that constitutes a food with little nutrient density, or we say lots of empty calories. Those foods with lots of empty calories are going to make their way through your digestive system faster and leave you feeling empty and wanting to eat more. It is like comparing a whole grain bagel to a doughnut. The bagel is going to stay with you longer even though they may have a comparable number of calories.

<u>What are Nutrient Poor Foods?</u>
Generally, the more processed a food is, the more nutrient poor a food becomes. Just look at white flour. When wheat is milled, the bran and germ are taken off leaving the endosperm. The endosperm is white with many of the nutrients removed. This was first done to preserve shelf-life. But removing components for the sake of shelf-life also removes valuable nutrients. White flour is so processed that bugs won't eat it. Now, they do add back some of the nutrients that are lost in processing. This is called enriching, but what about the nutrients that are not put back? Look at the fiber content for instance. They do not add back fiber and fiber is severely lacking in most Americans' diets. And what about all the nutrients that we may not know about yet? Goodness knows, for all the research that has been done we still can't make a carrot.

If you stick with mostly whole foods, you are likely to get the most nutrients in your diet and the most variety of nutrients in your diet. Now, they also do something called fortification. That is, the manufacturers add nutrients that were not originally there. But again, they can only do this with the nutrients that we currently know, using the information about those nutrients that we currently have. The amounts and ratios of those nutrients may not prove to be ideal.

The easiest way to think of the nutrient poor foods is to think of those foods that are: White. I know we covered these foods previously (white flour, pasta, rice, and sugars). They were something our ancestors didn't have or had in very limited supply, and the more you can incorporate whole grains rather than white grains, the more satisfying and nutrient dense your diet can be.

<u>Eating in America</u>

Now I know I listed a ton of foods that are the bad guys, and I am sure you are thinking you can't do without a few of them. But wait before you start to get discouraged and let's think about a few things first. We live in a fat nation. "Results from the 1999-2002 National Health and Nutrition Examination Survey (NHANES), using measured heights and weights, indicate that an estimated 65 percent of U.S. adults are either overweight or obese. This represents a prevalence that is 16 percent higher than the overweight estimates from 1988-94." [60] We, as a nation, are fat and getting fatter. I am sure you want to be one of the ones who is lean, fit, and healthy. In July of 2007, the United States population was estimated at 301 million.[61] This means that there were about 180 million overweight people in the U.S.

854 million people across the world are hungry,[62] with a world population estimated at 6,602 million (6.6 billion).[63] If you take the ratio of hungry people in the world to overweight people in the U.S., the ratio is about one-third. That means in theory that if the U.S. population got to a good weight, we could eliminate a third of the world's hunger. Well, you know that isn't exactly true, because we know that hunger has more

---

[60] "Prevalence of Overweight and Obesity among Adults: United States, 1999-2002." U.S. DEPARTMENT OF HEALTH AND HUMAN SERVICES, Centers for Disease Control and Prevention, National Center for Health Statistics, Hyattsville, MD 20782. www.cdc.gov/nchs/products/pubs/pubd/hestats/obese/obse99.htm
[61] "World Fact Book: United States." https://www.cia.gov/library/publications/the-world-factbook/print/us.html
[62] State of Food Insecurity in the World 2006. Food and Agriculture Organization of the United Nations. 2006.
[63] "World Fact Book: World." https://www.cia.gov/library/publications/the-world-factbook/print/xx.html

causes than just a simple lack of food, like politics and war, but it is something interesting to think about. Here we are, with most of our population overweight and obese, when there are 854 million people out there hungry, thirteen percent of the world's population, or more than one in ten people. Goodness knows there are people right here in the U.S. that are hungry or at risk of going hungry.

We are so lucky to be American. We have food to eat. But the truth is that our food supply is making us sick, just as a lack of food is making other people sick in other parts of the world, under different conditions. Just because we have food to eat, doesn't mean that it is good food or the right food to eat. It just means that food is readily available in our food supply. In fact, low income populations are at risk of being overweight or obese.

When they released the weight loss drug Orlistat (Xenical) as an over-the-counter drug, one hundred-twenty, 60mg pills, cost $69.99. Taken three times a day with meals as directed, this will cost $1.75 a day. Orlistat is formulated to bind fat in the gut, keep it from being absorbed, and send it out with the rest of the stool. Fat malabsorption is called steatorrhea, or fatty stool. This is a sign of poor absorption and a sign that something is wrong. You can recognize it by fat floating on the water after you have a bowel movement. What kind of crazy marketing came up with the idea to let you be able to spend more money on eating fat and paying for a drug to get you to poop it out? Why not take the $1.75 a day and eat a little less fat yourself and donate the rest to help feed some of those hungry people we mentioned rather than just eating it and wasting it?!? Turns out, this drug has not had much of a following. Having steatorrhea is not a very pleasant sensation and most people can't tolerate it for very long.

Most of the world is vegetarian most of the time. That means there is a huge variety of foods to cook and eat. Americans eat only a few basic foods most of the time. By adding vegetarian foods, you add a huge array of foods from a world of cuisines. The trick is to eat a variety of foods that are nutrient dense and appeal to you..

<u>How Do I Get Nutrient Dense Foods?</u>
Here is a quick list to give you some ideas about what to eat. These are just some of the great vegetarian foods that are high in nutritional value – and that is what you want. Don't worry if this seems complicated – just eat a variety of foods using this guide to give you some ideas. Eat what you like and try new foods.

Now I know it will seem like a lot, but this will give you two things. One is a list of nutrients so when you are asked: "Where do you get your this," you can say what it is found in and what you are eating. Second is the knowledge that most foods contain numerous nutrients and by eating a variety of foods, you will have all of your nutrient bases covered. Get ready. You are about to become a vegan nutrient pro.

- <u>Eat Foods High in Protein.</u> Protein is needed for building muscles and restoring your organs. Some great sources of protein include beans, soy like tofu, tempeh, TVP (texturized vegetable protein), soy milks, fake meats, nuts (like almonds, Brazil nuts, cashews, hazel nuts, peanuts, pine nuts), seeds (like flax seeds, pumpkin seeds, sesame seeds, sunflower seeds), legumes (like dried peas, beans, and lentils), and grains, cereals, and pasta like those made from whole wheat, barley, rye, oats, millet, corn, and rice. Don't be worried about eating any special combination of proteins, just eat a variety of them. They used to say that you had to combine certain proteins at meal to get all you needed. Now, it is widely recognized that the body has an "amino acid pool" and that certain amino acids, or pieces of protein, will combine to form proteins as your body needs them.

- <u>Eat some Good Carbohydrates.</u> Carbohydrates should be your major source of energy. Try whole grains like whole wheat, oats, barley, rice, whole-wheat bread, whole grain pastas, and other flour products, lentils, beans, potatoes, dried and fresh fruit, and lots of vegetables.

- <u>Eat some good Quality Fats</u> that provide the essential fatty acids. The two polyunsaturated fatty acids that you need that are not made by the body are linoleic acid, the omega 6s, and alpha-linolenic acid, the omega 3s.   Eat a variety of nuts and seeds, plant, nut, and seed oils, nonhydrogenated (no trans-fat) margarine, or avocados. Eat good sources of Linoleic Acid (Omega-6) like safflower, sunflower, corn, evening primrose, or soy oils, and eat good sources of Alpha-linolenic Acid (Omega-3) like flaxseed, pumpkin seed, walnut, soy, and canola oils. I also include olive oil for sure as a source of monounsaturated fatty acids. You can use it in salads or cooking, including baking, as the Greeks do. More and more research is linking it to longevity.

- Eat a variety of these foods for plenty of health-giving <u>Water-Soluble Vitamins</u> (vitamins that dissolve in water) including:

- For Vitamin C: Eat plenty of fruit and vegetables including collard greens, broccoli, Brussels sprouts, oranges, lemons, limes, currants, tangerines, grapefruit, spinach, strawberries, green peppers, tomatoes, cantaloupe, berries, and potatoes.

- For Thiamin (Vitamin B1): Eat a variety of whole grain breads and cereals, wheat germ, sunflower seeds, peanuts, legumes.

- For Vitamin B2 (Riboflavin): Try whole grains, mushrooms, almonds, leafy green vegetables, and yeast extracts.

- For Niacin (Vitamin B3): Try peanuts, whole grains and cereals, peas, and Brewer's yeast.

- For Vitamin B6: Try bananas, lentils, wheat germ,

lentils, whole grains, oatmeal, cabbage.

- For Folate: Have some dark green leafy vegetables including spinach and collard greens, broccoli, legumes, peanuts and other nuts like almonds or cashews, wheat germ, yeast, yeast nutritional extracts, peas, green beans, oranges, dates, avocados, and whole grains.

- For Biotin: Eat a variety of foods since it is widely available, especially whole grain cereals, soybeans, yeast. It is also produced in abundance by bacteria in the intestine.

- For Pantothenic Acid: Eat a variety of foods since it is widely available especially grains and legume. It is produced by bacteria in the intestine as well.

- For Vitamin B12: Eat a variety of fortified soy, rice, and nut milks, TVP products, breakfast cereals, veggie-burger mixes, nutritional yeast extracts, seaweeds, and fermented soy products like tamari, miso and tempeh. B12 may also be produced in the intestine. You can also easily take a B12 supplement or make sure that it is in your multi-vitamin. This is really the one nutrient that used to be hard to get in a vegan diet, but now is readily available in the food supply. Cases of B12 deficiency are normally seen in those with digestive absorption problems such as the elderly who often get B12 shots. Cases were seen in the infants of vegan mothers who did not breastfeed their infants and gave non-formula milks. So remember, human breastmilk is for human babies. Moms breastfeed your babies! They'll love you for it by being healthier and smarter their whole lives. For the rest of us, make sure B12 is in the processed foods that you do eat such as soy milk or take B12 as a precaution in supplement form since a deficiency will cause nerve problems in the long run.

- Eat a variety of these foods for plenty of health-giving <u>Fat-Soluble Vitamins</u> (vitamins that dissolve in fat – yes, you do have to eat some fat):

- For Vitamin A: Eat dark green and dark orange foods including Brussels sprouts, spinach, collard greens, broccoli, carrots, peaches, apricots, tomatoes, pumpkin, and cantaloupe, fortified soy, rice, and nut milks, and nonhydrogenated margarines.
- For Vitamin D: Eat a variety of fortified soy, rice, and nut milks, and nonhydrogenated margarines. Vitamin D is also produced by sunlight on the skin.
- For Vitamin E: Try a variety of nuts, seeds like sunflower seeds, whole grains and flours, and vegetable oils.
- For Vitamin K: Try some leafy green vegetables, corn and soybean oil, whole grain cereals, and fruit.
- Also, eat a variety of these <u>MacroMinerals</u> (minerals needed in relatively large amounts).
- Eat foods high in Calcium. Calcium helps provide the structure of bones and teeth, and is involved in nerve impulse transmission, blood clotting, and muscle contraction. Eat a variety of nuts, seeds, soybeans, tofu, miso, molasses, carob, parsley, dried figs, sea vegetables, grains including oatmeal, fortified orange juice, and fortified soy and nut milks.
- Eat foods high in Iron. Iron helps transport oxygen as part of hemoglobin in blood and myoglobin in muscles, and it functions in electron transport. Eat a variety of nuts, seeds, beans, legumes, grains, dried fruit, sea vegetables, parsley, green leafy vegetables, molasses, and miso.
- Eat foods high in Zinc. Zinc is part of over 70 enzymes including those involved in growth, sexual maturation, fertility and reproduction, night vision, taste acuity, and immune function. Try eating

wheat germ, whole grains like whole wheat bread, rice, and oats, nuts, pulses, tofu, soy protein, miso, peas, parsley, bean sprouts, and alfalfa sprouts.

- Eat foods high in these <u>Trace Minerals</u> (minerals needed in relatively small amounts), too:
- Chromium: Chromium is involved in blood sugar function and again is found in whole grains, fruits, and vegetables including broccoli, potatoes, green beans, apples bananas, and grapes.
- Copper: Copper changes iron absorption and metabolism, and it is involved in many different enzymes. You can get it in nuts and seeds, leafy greens, chocolate, and mushrooms.
- Iodine: Iodine is part of thyroid gland hormones. Sources of iodine include seaweeds, vegetables, grains, prunes, and of course iodized salt.
- Magnesium: Magnesium is involved in over 300 enzyme systems. It can be found especially in whole grains, spinach, almonds, cashews, peanuts, chocolate, soy, avocado.
- Manganese and Molybdenum: Manganese and Molybdenum are involved in many enzymes. Manganese is in nuts including almonds and pecans, beans including lima and pinto beans, legumes, whole wheat, brown rice, dark greens, fruits like pineapple, and chocolate. Molybdenum is found in legumes like peas and lentils, beans like kidney, navy, and lima beans, nuts like almonds, chestnuts, cashews, and peanuts, soy, leafy greens, and whole grains.
- Phosphorus: Phosphorus functions as part of nucleic acids (DNA and RNA), helps form cell membranes, changes calcium concentrations, and helps keep acid and base in balance. It is found in many fruits and vegetables, whole grains, soy, nuts, and seeds.

- Selenium: Selenium is a scavenger for free radicals and therefore may help reduce the signs of aging. Brazil nuts and mushrooms are particularly high in selenium. It is also found in many beans and seeds.

If you are feeling overwhelmed right about now, please don't be. You have just received all you need to know about vegan nutrition. You don't need to memorize anything. You don't even have to know how to say everything. The point is just look over the list above to get ideas about what to eat and eat a variety of foods. Don't get in the habit of severely restricting yourself as far as the variety of foods that you eat. Be sure to eat an array of fruits, whole grains, nuts, seeds, and vegetables.

To get all you need nutritionally, this is your number one rule: Eat a variety of foods. Don't get stuck into the rut of eating the same things all the time. Variety is the spice of life and it helps keep you interested, satisfied, and motivated.

Why Do We Binge?

I told you about the donkeys we had growing up. Animals seem to know what to eat and, for the most part, what's good for them. For instance, rats don't become "obese" in nature, but they do become "obese" if you put them on a human junk food diet. Some researchers call this a supermarket diet. This seems to be the case with most animals. In the wild, they know what is good for them, but the domesticated ones eat what we do and may get too fat.

Also, in the wild, animals will binge and gorge. Animals after a kill will gorge. Primates will gorge on whatever fruit is ripe, just as human children might have sat under the grape arbor or under the apple tree and stuffed themselves. The problem is: There aren't too many of those grape arbors and apple trees anymore. This is the way our ancestors lived though. Whatever food was around, they ate a lot of and/or had to preserve for later use. It is much more natural to binge on whatever fruit is in season, than to binge on Halloween candy. And candy isn't only a Halloween thing anymore.

Food manufacturers purposely manufacture foods to make you want to eat more. Why would they want to make a food that you could have a handful of and be satisfied? They make foods to stimulate the appetite. These appetite stimulating foods may include salt, fat, sugar, yeast extracts, alcohol, and a host of food additives. These are put in foods to make them more appealing than they ever would be in nature. Bet you can't eat just one, right? They want you to eat more and the more they can pack that food with cheap ingredients, the better.

The simple truth is: Maybe some of us, at least, shouldn't eat these "foods" at all. Studies show that certain food acts in our brains to stimulate pleasure centers the same way illegal drugs stimulate, and addict, the brains of an addict by affecting dopamine. Sugar causes a dopamine response increasing its release in the nucleus accumbens of the brain. Studies have shown that if rats are dependent on sugar they will have delayed satiation, drink more sugar, and release more dopamine. Daily binging makes it worse.[64] Most drugs of abuse increase dopamine in the nucleus accumbens.[65] Daily sugar can also lead to a "pattern of excessive intake" and alterations in how both dopamine and opioids react in the brain, thus desensitizing the receptors that bind them.[66] Is it any wonder eating a lot of sugar just makes you want to eat more? In fact, experiments show that abstinence doesn't necessarily work either. After abstinence, you may actually be driven to eat more sugar than before just like other addictive drugs.[67] Fat consumption stimulates dopamine as well. The

---

[64] P.Radaab N.M.Avenaa B.G.Hoebela. Daily bingeing on sugar repeatedly releases dopamine in the accumbens shell. Neuroscience. Volume 134, Issue 3, 2005, Pages 737-744

[65] Ibid.

[66] Colantuoni, C.; Schwenker, J.; McCarthy, J.; Rada, P.; Ladenheim, B.; Cadet, J.-L.; Schwartz, G. J.; Moran, T. H.; Hoebel, B. G. Excessive sugar intake alters binding to dopamine and mu-opioid receptors in the brain. NeuroReport: November 16th, 2001 - Volume 12 - Issue 16 - p 3549-3552

[67] Nicole M.AvenaKristin A.LongBartley G.Hoebel.Sugar-dependent rats

overconsumption of fat is thought to actually decrease the sensitivity of this dopamine-reward sensation and lead to an even greater fat consumption. The mechanism for this is unclear,[68] but the greater the BMI in humans the less the availability of dopamine (D_2) receptors.[69]

If you want to get an idea of what life used to be like, get a farm share from a local farmer. Each week during growing season you will get what is in season. This is one of the principal components of macrobiotics: eat what is in season in your area. Binge eating disorder is a real thing that we will talk about later, but the truth is that all of us have some tendency to gorge on occasion. If, however, you eat what is in season, there is new evidence that what you eat may actually be beneficial. For example, peaches have polyphenolics that have been shown to act as an anti-cancer agent. They have been shown to inhibit tumor growth and metastasis of breast cancer cells.[70] Peaches are never in season in one location all the time and you need a large dose of some of these natural anti-cancer compounds to have an effect. There are all kinds of other similar examples in the plant kingdom of chemopreventive and anticancer phytochemicals. Perhaps, we were meant to gorge on peaches on occasion to get our dose of polyphenolics to act as a medicinal against cancer. So, next time you're thinking

---

show enhanced responding for sugar after abstinence: Evidence of a sugar deprivation effect Physiology & Behavior
Volume 84, Issue 3, 16 March 2005, Pages 359-362.
[68] Luis A. Tellez, Sara Medina, Wenfei Han, Jozelia G. Ferreira, Paula Licona-Limón. A Gut Lipid Messenger Links Excess Dietary Fat to Dopamine Deficiency. Science 16 Aug 2013: Vol. 341, Issue 6147, pp. 800-802, DOI: 10.1126/science.1239275
[69] DrGene-JackWang,MD, Nora DVolkowMD, JeanLoganPhD, Naoml RPappasMS, Christopher TWongCNMT, WelZhuPhD, NoelwahNetusllRN, Joanna SFowlerPhD. Brain dopamine and obesity The Lancet. Volume 357, Issue 9253, 3 February 2001, Pages 354-357.
[70] GiulianaNoratto, WestonPorter, DavidByrne, LuisCisneros-Zevallos. Polyphenolics from peach (Prunus persica var. Rich Lady) inhibit tumor growth and metastasis of MDA-MB-435 breast cancer cells in vivo. The Journal of Nutritional Biochemistry. Volume 25, Issue 7, July 2014, Pages 796-800.

about eating a lot of something, and not feeling guilty, try thinking about what is in season and abundant in your local growing area. Chances are, what's in abundance at the farmers' market this week is not going to break your diet, and perhaps, it might even be very good for you.

Kind verses Quantity.

There are two main approaches to dieting: Selecting different kinds of foods and selecting different quantities of foods. Chances are that you have had a great deal of experience with the later. Most diet programs rely on reducing the quantity of the food you eat. You have to start measuring what you eat, counting servings per day, or only eating what comes in your monthly food package in the mail. Lowering the quantity of what you eat in my estimation is the much harder method. First off, if you are overweight, you are probably used to eating too much of everything. Your stomach is about the size of a quart of milk. Any more than this causes several things to happen. For one thing, the stomach stretches. When this happens, you can eat more, it takes longer for you to feel full, you get used to this feeling, and you perpetually eat too much. Another thing that can happen when you eat too much is that the food already in your stomach gets pushed out the other end into the small intestine. This is okay in that you can thus eat more, but not all right because the food that gets pushed out is not digested as well as it should be. The stomach contains strong acid to break down the food you eat. Without enough exposure to this acid, food pushed down the digestive tract will not have the nutrients it contains broken down and absorbed properly. It also leaves substances in the digestive tract that bacteria down the system can fester in creating gas and all kinds of abdominal pain and other issues. Lastly, if you eat too much the food can work its way back up the esophagus. After all, there are only so many places it can go. This can cause stomach upset, heart burn, and reflux. The lining of the esophagus can actually erode. Also, if you really have overdone it sometime, this can lead to vomiting.

Most diet programs ask you to reduce the quantity of what you eat. If you are used to being full, this can be a major use of willpower. Willpower for eating smaller amounts has been shown to decrease due to stress and later in the day. We seem to only have a certain amount of willpower to spare and then it can be used up. Have you ever noticed that if you had a very stressful day, the diet is just shot? This can happen over the course of a single day or a week. Have you ever been good for a week and then just blew it? That's why. And we never seem to blow-it with healthy foods, do we? Most diet programs ask you to add your own fresh items to their diet foods. You must add produce and diary, right? It is very easy to add too much in the way of sweet yogurts and cheeses, right? Adding to your diet program can blow it. It is very easy to eat all your foods for the day and still be hungry. Being hungry is hard. Sometimes the temptation to eat all your pre-packaged desserts for the week is just too much.

The other way to go is to change the kind of food you eat. Vegan food is the healthiest way to go. You can fill yourself up and not feel guilty. If you decide to eat lots of eggs and dairy, you'll still be having lots of calories, so it is best to try to cut these out as well. Far better to eat a lot of most any vegetarian/vegan food than most any animal product. Not only are animal products higher in fat and calories, but they also tend to be cooked in some very unhealthy ways. Deep frying anything though isn't doing yourself a favor. As long as you are improving the kinds of foods you are eating, please try to pick the healthiest methods of preparation you can. I would also recommend not overdoing it on fatty foods like nuts or avocadoes. These foods are good in moderation, but if you eat too much, not only will you be eating a bunch of fat and calories, but you may suffer the discomfort of having them sit in your stomach a long time, too. Fat can take a long time to digest.

The other thing that eating strictly vegan food will do for you is to help you avoid some of the worse foods for weight loss: all those white foods I mentioned above. If you take the time to look at an ingredient list to see what is in that cake or cookie before you eat it, it gives you another chance to think about if you really want to eat it. Seeing that it contains milk or eggs is an easy, instant way to tell yourself to put it down. I also tell people to skip things with ingredients that you don't know what they are, or you don't know where they came from. Some people say: "Don't eat foods with ingredients you can't pronounce." The more you get to study these ingredients, the more you find that you don't consider many of these things to be foods. The more you learn that many of these products are derived from petroleum products, come from rocks, or are so highly processed (often in other chemicals that are later removed) so much that you would not consider them food, you may not want to eat them. For a good book on this subject, read *Twinkie, Deconstructed* by Steve Ettlinger for an entertaining, informative look at where the ingredients found in a Twinkie, and many other foods, come from.

Why Would You Want to Do Anything So Radical?

I've heard it said before, and I'm sure you will too, "Why would you want to anything so radical as become a vegetarian, worse yet, a vegan? Don't you miss meat (cheese, eggs)?"

Well, let's consider the alternative. First, you could stay overweight. Most likely, you would gain at least a couple of pounds a year, like most Americans, and get heavier. With increased weight comes increased risk of disease and disability, or worsening conditions if your unfortunate enough to have them already. With increased illness comes increased medication, and on the cycle goes, more illness, more medication, more side effects, more doctor visits, and more medical costs.

Second, you've tried other radical things already. You probably have starved yourself or exercised until you were so sore you gave up or ate some crazy diet that made you feel sick or was just as dangerous to do long-term or purged in one way or another. You might have taken medications (and suffered their side effect) or even had surgery. You may even have been told by your doctor to gain a few more pounds because you were not eligible yet for gastric bypass surgery, but if you gained a few more pounds your insurance would cover it. This sounds radical to me. I can't imagine telling a patient to gain more weight when weight gain is obviously detrimental to their overall health.

Let's consider gastric bypass surgery for a moment. Gastric bypass surgery is touted by the media as being a miracle for people who have tried everything. Advertisers portrait it as glamourous. There are real, serious complication, however, including death that may result. You may suffer hemorrhage, wound complications, leakage, deep venous thrombophlebitis, pulmonary embolism, and pneumonia during hospitalization. After hospitalization you are at risk for protein malnutrition, deficiencies of vitamins A, B1, B12, D, K, and folate, and the minerals iron, zinc, calcium, copper, and selenium and the complications arising from these deficiencies. You may suffer steatorrhea (floating fatty diarrhea), dumping syndrome (rapid heartbeat and low blood pressure after eating high-sugar foods experienced by about seventy-five percent of patients), anastomotic stricture or ulceration, internal or ventral hernias, bowel obstruction, fistulas, cholelithiasis (gallstones), islet cell hypertrophy, gastric band slippage and, after all that, insufficient weight loss to boot.[71] Fifteen to seventeen percent of patients fail to lose even two-fifths to fifty percent of their excess weight. So, if for instance you need to lose one hundred pounds, almost two out of ten people won't even lose 40 to 50 pounds. That means they would still be fifty to six pounds overweight. On top of that you will have to take a vitamin and mineral supplement the rest of your life which must include daily calcium, B12, folic acid, and zinc plus iron three times daily.[72] Without supplementation, patients develop deficiency

---

[71] Cleek, John B., Westman, Eric C. "Surgical Treatment of the obese individual," Obesity: Evaluation and Treatment Essentials, Second Edition. G.Michael Steelman, Eric C. Westman, eds. CRC Press, New York, 2016.
[72] Ibid.

diseases. You'll also have to make sure that you never eat too much at a time or risk vomiting and diarrhea. Patients who fail to lose weight or regain weight are more likely to be sedentary, eat fast food, continue eating when full, eat continuously, binge eat or lose control eating, and weigh themselves less than once week, all behaviors that helped make them overweight in the first place. Patients with less weight loss are also more likely to be younger, have venous edema (swollen limbs due to venous insufficiency), poorer physical function, and more depression.[73] I would rather try to change some of my behaviors than undergo surgery and then have to try changing my behaviors anyway. Surgery could be a lot of unnecessary suffering.

The same goes for liposuction. Liposuction is not considered a treatment for obesity. It is portrayed so glamorously in the media, yet it is so ineffective in reality. Since fat cells are removed, fat is deposited in untreated areas of the body (including visceral fat around the organs further increasing your risk of heart disease and diabetes) and remaining fat cells. Liposuction, along with tummy tucks and body lifting to remove excess skin, are considered body contouring, that is reshaping, not effective means of weight loss.

With the other solutions out there harboring such risk and pain, and ineffectiveness, how is giving up meat something so radical? Sounds to me like it's an easy thing to try. It might even be fun learning to eat new foods, learning new recipes, and getting a new lease on life.

<u>The Deficiency Diseases of the Overweight and Obese.</u>
We think of obesity as being a condition of excess and yet ironically, malnutrition exists in obesity. In fact, it is the very deficiencies of obesity that might make diabetes more prevalent. Vitamin D deficiency is present in as much as 80 to

---

[73] King WC, Belle SH, Hinerman AS, Mitchell JE, Steffen KJ, Courcoulas AP. Patient Behaviors and Characteristics Related to Weight Regain After Roux-en-Y Gastric Bypass: A Multicenter Prospective Cohort Study. Ann Surg. 2019 Apr 4.

90 percent of the obese.[74] Vitamin D, chromium, biotin, thiamine (B1), and vitamin C all play a role in diabetes and may be compromised in obese individuals. Studies show that the obese have a prevalence of 15 to 29 percent for thiamine deficiency, up to eleven percent for pyridoxine (B6) deficiency, up to eight percent for B12 deficiency, 35 to 45 percent for vitamin C deficiency, 17 percent for vitamin A deficiency, 14 to 30 percent for zinc deficiency, and 58 percent for selenium deficiency.[75] Our all-American diet seems to be keeping us fat, but not well-fed. It doesn't seem to me that becoming vegan

[74] Kaidar-Person O, Person B, Szomstein S, Rosenthal RJ. Nutritional deficiencies in morbidly obese patients: a new form of malnutrition? Part A: vitamins. Obesity Surgery. 2008;18(7):870–876.
Strohmayer E, Via MA, Yanagisawa R. Metabolic management following bariatric surgery. Mount Sinai Journal of Medicine. 2010;77(5):431–445.
[75] Kaidar-Person O, Person B, Szomstein S, Rosenthal RJ. Nutritional deficiencies in morbidly obese patients: a new form of malnutrition? Part A: vitamins. Obesity Surgery. 2008;18(7):870–876.
Kaidar-Person O, Person B, Szomstein S, Rosenthal RJ. Nutritional deficiencies in morbidly obese patients: a new form of malnutrition? Part B: minerals. Obesity Surgery. 2008;18(8):1028–1034.
Ekmekcioglu C, Prohaska C, Pomazal K, Steffan I, Schernthaner G, Marktl W. Concentrations of seven trace elements in different hematological matrices in patients with type 2 diabetes as compared to healthy controls. Biological Trace Element Research. 2001;79(3):205–219.
Coupaye M, Puchaux K, Bogard C, et al. Nutritional consequences of adjustable gastric banding and gastric bypass: a 1-year prospective study. Obesity Surgery. 2009;19(1):56–65.
Pflipsen MC, Oh RC, Saguil A, Seehusen DA, Topolski R. The prevalence of vitamin B12 deficiency in patients with type 2 diabetes: a cross-sectional study. Journal of the American Board of Family Medicine. 2009;22(5):528–534.
de Luis DA, Pacheco D, Izaola O, Terroba MC, Cuellar L, Martin T. Clinical results and nutritional consequences of biliopancreatic diversion: three years of follow-up. Annals of Nutrition and Metabolism. 2008;53(3-4):234–239.
Gehrer S, Kern B, Peters T, Christofiel-Courtin C, Peterli R. Fewer nutrient deficiencies after laparoscopic sleeve gastrectomy (LSG) than after Laparoscopic Roux-Y-gastric bypass (LRYGB)-a prospective study. Obesity Surgery. 2010;20(4):447–453.

would be giving anything up. Becoming vegan may be just what we need to become better nourished.

<u>Let's Get Some Ideas on Our New Road to Health.</u>
When you are first starting out on any new diet, you really may have no idea of what to eat. Thing if it this way: "You learned to cook one way. Vegan is just another way to cook." If you wanted to cook fine French cuisine, you might feel lost in the beginning, too. What you really need is some ideas.

One of the best ways to get ideas is going to a vegetarian potluck. Vegetarian and vegan groups have sprung up all over the country. All you have to do is do a search the internet to find one. A lot of vegetarian groups have potlucks on a regular basis. I know ours does. Check a few out. Not only will you get some good ideas for what to eat, but you'll get a good sampling of dishes to try so you see what you like without having to make every recipe in your cookbook. You'll also meet some great people and hopefully learn a lot in the process, too.

If you do a simple search on the internet for vegetarian or vegan recipes, look at the images. By looking at photos you'll know what looks appetizing to you and get great ideas for meals using techniques you know how to do already. The beauty of much of vegetarian cooking is that you don't need a recipe. After you get an idea of what to make, recipes can be extremely flexible. After all, do you really need to know just how much broccoli to put in your stir-fry or how many beans to put in your burrito? Save the recipes for baking when it matters more if the "chemistry" of the recipe is right.

In the meantime, what you really need is ideas. Try to eliminate animal products whenever you can. For now, here are some ideas of what to eat at different meals that may help when you are first starting out.

For breakfast, you could try:
- Oatmeal with soy or rice milk
- Pancakes or waffles made with whole grain flour
- Fresh fruit
- A protein shake

For lunch, you could try:
- A vegetarian deli slice sandwich
- Tofu salad
- Bean salad
- Veggie hot dogs

For dinner, you might try:
- A bean burrito or taco
- A veggie burger
- A stir-fry
- Lentil soup
- Whole grain pasta

For snacks, try:
- Cut-up vegetables
- Fresh fruit
- Marinated tofu (tofu with soy sauce, spices, and vinegar or your choice)
- Whole grain toast
- Nuts

So, here is the deal. Eat life-giving foods. For the most part that means that if you planted them, they might grow. This means vegetables, fruits, whole grain, beans, legumes, and the minimally processed foods made from them. Here are some more ideas.

<u>What's for Breakfast?</u>

As Americans we tend to think of a limited number of foods for breakfast, but there is really no reason for this. Other cultures might have rice, noodles, or vegetables for -breakfast. You could have last-night's leftovers. For breakfast you might try fruit, whole grain cereal or toast. You could have a salad or a handful of nuts. You could have a homemade muffin or a bowl of oatmeal. A lot of people are in a hurry so grabbing something is just fine, just make sure it is healthy.

Here is a trick: Put healthy foods where you can see them. Far better to be tempted by a bowl of apples and bananas than a plastic pack of store-bought muffins. Most of the traditional American breakfast foods have a way of making you feel terrible later in the morning. The muffins, croissants, pancakes, waffles, toast and jelly, pastries, and the like, have a way of making me feel comatose not too long afterwards. Here's what happens if I eat them. I'm tired and groggy from a poor night's sleep; this might typically happen at a hotel, because I don't ever do this to myself at home. The muffins or pancakes look good, so I take one. One turns into some. They are definitely not whole grain (even if they look brown). They will have fake-maple syrup and I'll eat more because they taste good and everyone else is eating too and I want to be social. Besides, I'm waiting for everyone else to finish. The food is not only sweet, it is fatty, and before I come to my senses knowing that I never should have started this nonsense, I feel sick in the stomach. Sugar has a way of doing that to a lot of people. The sugar is what they call hydrophilic and pulls water into the digestive system causing cramps. I feel kind of hyper, but then I feel cranky, even though I'm supposed to be having fun. Later I get tired, then still later I feel like I might just pass out. An argument may even ensue. Well, my research says that a lot of people feel this way. The thing is though that most people think this is the way they are supposed to feel – tired and barely able to make it though they day.

Eating a junky, refined carbohydrate/sugary, fatty breakfast leaves you in the position of eating this kind of food all day long. The sugar is high in your blood, but the body more than compensates leaving you with blood sugar that is too low. This leaves you craving fatty, sugary foods the rest of the day. This kind of eating leaves your body unable to regulate your caloric needs. They used to say that children up to five years old perfectly regulated what they intake on a daily basis so that their caloric intake barely varies. They are not saying this anymore. That is because people used to feed their children a diet based on whole foods with very little processed convenience foods. Most people don't anymore. They have junky, processed foods from the beginning of the day to the end.

When you don't eat whole unprocessed foods, you lose your ability to regulate your intake, regardless of your age. As I have said before, when they give this kind of diet to lab mice,[76] they call it the "supermarket diet" and mice can't regulate their caloric intake either. Salt, sugar, fat, and the host of other junk they add make it taste too good, and the lack of bulk make it so you can eat endlessly without feeling full, so that if you do this on any regular basis you will gain weight.

Refined sugar and white flour are essentially digested and absorbed immediately upon ingestion. Yes, you must chew them and swallow them and break them down just a little bit in the stomach, but this is essentially like hooking yourself up to an IV of glucose, because the sugar is headed straight for your veins. It also leaves essentially nothing left behind in the stomach to make you feel full. There is nothing left in there, so you can eat for a longer period of time or want to eat another meal soon because the last meal didn't leave you without anything to digest. This is called a low-residue diet and it is used as a means of leaving less in the digestive system before a diagnostic procedure on the bowel or in the acute stages of certain chronic bowel illnesses such as bowel obstruction. A low residue diet consists of refined white flour products, white

---

[76] Mind you, I'm against the use of animals in experimentation, but that is a topic for another day.

rice, fruit juice without pulp, bananas and melons, canned fruit, skinless potato products, canned vegetables, well-cooked meat, milk products, oil, margarine, and butter. Laxatives are often prescribed with this diet to clean out the colon. Except for bananas and melons, this is not how you want to eat for weight-loss or long-term health. The diet that most Americans eat is pretty similar to a low-residue diet. The problem is though that all the marketing trying to make a difference on this subject is focused on the "dreadful fiber." Who among us does not think of our grandmother's laxative cereal or dry, rock-hard bran muffins? The fiber that is good for us is not the dry additive, by-product of food processing. The fiber that is good for us is that which is contained in whole foods naturally. That dry, boxed stuff is not the life-giving stuff you want. You want the whole fruits, vegetable, whole grains, beans, and legumes that have it in them naturally and don't need added fiber to make them appear healthy. I hope I've made the case that the big, hotel breakfast is not what you want, and I didn't even talk about all the normal pork products people eat. You want something healthy and don't worry if someone else might eat it for lunch or dinner and think it weird to have for breakfast; it really doesn't matter. Healthy food is healthy food no matter the time of day.

Here some things I like for breakfast that don't leave me falling asleep: any kind of fresh fruit, a handful of nuts with an apple, peanut butter on a cut-up apple, a mug of hot tea maybe with a little unsweetened soy milk or oat milk, last night's leftovers, oatmeal with cinnamon and nutmeg or mace, whole grain crackers, or tofu cubes with a little soy sauce.

And if you want a big shot of healthy, whole grain fiber and healthy, omega-3 fatty acids, try this: fresh, hot flax seed cereal. If I had a restaurant (which I might someday), I'd call it "The Regular." Flax seeds are often used as an egg-substitute in baking because they make a rather slimy, gelatinous layer when mixed with water and bind the baked good together. I wouldn't call this idea "slimy," I'd call it smooth. The longer is sits though, the thicker it will get, and it will bulk up your stools, something that you may want on occasion. For a healthier, fresher product, use freshly ground flax seeds. My mother-in-law got me an electric spice grinder one year and it makes the perfect flax seed cereal serving size for one.

Hot Flax Seed Cereal: For hot, fresh flax seed cereal, take fresh flax seeds and give them a whirl in the spice grinder. This should only take a few seconds. Put your ground flax seeds in a mug and cover with boiling, hot water and give it a stir. Let sit for a few minutes to cool before eating. Add more water for a porridge that you can drink, less water to eat it with a spoon. For fun additions, add spices like cinnamon, nutmeg, mace, allspice, or vanilla. Many herbs and spices have been shown to have anti-cancer and other health-giving properties. I add them whenever I can, fresh or dried. You only need a little to add a lot of flavor to your food. For another fun addition, try adding a small amount of dried fruit. I like raisins, currants, chopped figs, or dates. You can add them at the end or before adding your boiling water. Adding them beforehand, allows them to absorb water and digest more slowly while they fill your belly and draw water into your system. Hot flax cereal can be a comfort on a cold day.

<u>Lunch-time Ideas.</u>
Lunchtime is yet another time when we maybe short of time. We always seem to be running around anymore, don't we? That is no longer an excuse though for grabbing any old thing that is available and shoving it in your mouth while you're running off to the next thing or zoning-out in front of the computer, the TV, or your phone. A lot of times it is better just not to eat than eating something that you know is junk and is going to make you feel like crap latter. Sure, you could just grab some junk and eat less of it thinking that is going to help you lose weight. It is not going to help you in the long-term though. It takes more self-control than most people have available to eat just a small quantity of junk.

If you look for them, there a lot of healthy options out there, more so than there have ever been before. Most restaurants and even fast food places are trying to offer something healthy, sometimes even vegan. My rule is that what I do most of the time is what makes the difference in the long run; Doing something occasionally won't sink the ship. Afterall, any port in a storm; sometimes you just need to grab something. With this in mind, make yourself a list of things that you vow to yourself to never eat and those foods that you feel any port in a storm is good.

Foods I vow to never, ever eat:

____

____

____

____

Foods I will only eat if I am starving and nothing else is available:

____

____

____

____

<u>Dinner-time Ideas.</u>

For me, dinnertime is like lunchtime with the exception that I usually have more time for preparation. Here are some ideas for getting started.

Try some frozen food or an easy mix to get ideas of what you like. After you know the kinds of foods you like then you can spend more time learning to prepare them on your own to make them both healthier and less expensive. Frozen food and mixes tend to be high in salt, to say the least, and most of the time quite expensive especially if you are trying to feed multiple people.

Try "doctoring-up" some of your pre-prepared, store-bought salads and meals. For example, my husband loves store-bought chickpea salad and tabbouleh. Both are rather expensive and rather high in fat. Here is what I do, and by the way, I don't think he knows, my kids who help in the kitchen know though. I add one large can of chickpeas to the chickpea salad (just drain and rinse them with water first). Give it a stir and let it sit a few minutes before serving to let the flavors blend, and no one will ever know. I do the same thing with the tabbouleh by adding more diced tomatoes. Tomatoes are easy to add, but we can get parsley in the store quite inexpensively, too. Parsley is one of those things they tell you is related to decreased cancer.[77] I like chopping this up and throwing it in as well, just let it sit a while to let the flavors meld before serving.

My husband also likes frozen Indian food and those shelf-stable Indian food packets of curry and vegetable. When you by these, they turn out to be mostly sauce and not much else. I heat them on the stove and add appropriate things to make them healthier (less fat) and stretch them. Indian chickpeas (chana) can always take another can or two of chickpeas. Indian potato (aloo) dishes can always take a couple more boiled potatoes or left-over baked potatoes. Cut-up chunks of tofu also make a great, healthy, high-protein addition to Indian dishes. Crumbed tofu it also great to use instead of meat in those taco-mix kits you can buy. Drain the tofu, squish it through your fingers into a pot, and heat up with the mix and some water.

If you want to eat like some of the healthiest people in the world, the Ikarians of the Greek Island of Ikaria, have a bean-based salad. Bean salads are easy to make, especially if you use canned beans. Take a can of beans, any that you like, drain them and rinse them off. Add whatever chopped-up vegetables you like; I like onion or red onion, celery, and carrot. Add whatever spices you like; I like black pepper, always, and maybe some Italian spice or some dried vegetable blend. Give it a splash of vinegar (apple cider or red wine vinegar are great) and a splash of oil (flax seed, walnut, or extra virgin olive oil are great health-wise). Give it a toss and eat or let it sit a while to let the flavors meld.

---

[77] Guo Qiang. Zheng, Patrick M. Kenney, Luke K. T. Lam. Myristicin: a potential cancer chemopreventive agent from parsley leaf oil. J. Agric. Food Chem., 1992, 40 (1), pp 107–110.

Stir-fries are always a great, throw-together meal as well. These are especially easy if you have cooked rice on hand but remember you can make them on their own or over pasta as well. Always try to use brown rice and whole grain pasta for the added fiber and nutrients. Stir-fries are fun with a big pan or a wok if you have it. Chop-up a bunch of the vegetables you want to use before you get your pan going. When you're ready, heat your pan up and drizzle your oil down the edges of the pan in a circle to coat the whole pan. Start by adding the vegetables that you want cooked the most and progressively adding the softer vegetables that require less cooking and you don't want to get mushy. I usually start my stir-fries with onion or something like an onion, like a shallot or leek. I often add celery or carrots at this point as well. These vegetables will form the base and the flavor of your dish, so add what you like and change things up once in a while for variety. You can have a purely vegetable stir-fry, or my family likes when I add some tofu. If you add tofu, you can vary your dish by cooking the tofu anywhere from a crisp to soft and just hot. Tempeh, a kind of natural soy burger, is also great for stir-fries. You could add beans or dumplings, too. Later in cooking you'll want to add other vegetables that require less cooking such as broccoli, zucchini, or any leafy greens that just need a little bit of wilting, maybe even just stirred in at the very end. You can always add a sauce, too. Do this toward the end of cooking. My family likes a store-bought teriyaki sauce I buy. Just watch if you buy a sauce, don't use too much. These products are often laden with salt, sugar, and fat. When you find a sauce you like, read the ingredients and try to duplicate the ingredients on your own. They are usually very simple. Peanut butter in a sauce will give you more of a Thai flavor, soy will be more Chinese, red pepper flakes will give you a little punch. It you like your sauces a little on the thick side use a little corn starch (or for you purists, arrowroot powder). To use corn starch, remember that you must put corn starch in a little liquid to make a slurry before you add it to your dish, or you will be left with a lot of lumps. Also remember that corn starch must come to a boil to reach its full thickening potential. This is very easy to do in a stir fry. Add your sauce last, give it a stir, bring it to a boil (this will happen almost instantly with a very hot pan), and shut the heat off. Give it a few minutes to cool down and you're good to go. To give you an idea of a sauce we like, I take a heaping tablespoonful of corn starch in a cup, add a splash of water, a splash of soy sauce, maybe some chili flakes for a little heat, maybe a splash of vinegar for a little acidity, a tablespoon or two of peanut butter for Thai flavor, or a teaspoon or so of garlic granules, give it a good stir.[78] Add this mixture to your stir fry, and stir until just boiling and well thickened. In a hot wok, this could take less than a minute.

There are tons of vegetarian and vegan cookbooks out there. My cookbook is <u>One Hand Cooking: Vegetarian.</u> It came out in 2009 when my kids were little. I only ever had one hand to cook with at the time, because my other arm was always busy holding a kid on my hip. Yes, it is vegan, and you can see a cute picture of my kids on the cover.

<u>Going "Cold Turkey" or Taking "Baby Steps."</u>
A smoker who is going to quit makes the decision to cut down, little by little, week after week. Then something happens. Remember the "Airplane" movies? The pilot or air-traffic controller says something like: "Looks like I picked a bad week to quit drinking/ smoking/ sniffing glue!" just as something else horrible is happening with the airplane. Just when you quit, something else comes along to make it so you think you shouldn't have. There never seems to be a good time because something stressful always seems to come up. There never seems to be a good time to stop a bad habit, does there? That smoker who tries to cut down little by little, week after week is going to have a really hard time. It is very difficult to keep your conviction to only smoke one cigarette a day, when the rest of the pack is staring you in the face and you are under

---

[78] You need to mix corn starch with a little water before adding it to a larger amount of water or you will get lumps that are almost impossible to smooth out.

an inordinate amount of stress. Having only one cigarette a day may well be much more difficult than quitting altogether.

Going vegetarian or vegan can be the same way. Some people feel more control cutting out animal products altogether. On the other hand, some of the participant in my work said they switched to veganism over a long period of time and this made it easier. As they found more vegan foods they liked and got more healthy ideas, they missed the non-veggie foods less.

Certainly, the choice is up to you. It also depends on what and how much you are trying to accomplish. Maybe you don't ever want to have a doughnut, whatever they are made of, in the house again because you know if you buy them, they will disappear sooner or later. In my case, sooner.

Your motivation will also be influenced by your results. By weighing yourself regularly you should see results. Again, the more animal products you ate initially, the larger the reduction you will likely experience. Losing weight while feeling healthy is always great motivation.

<u>Making the Diet Work for You.</u>
Any steps toward veganism may be beneficial to you. The trick is making the diet your own and getting used to a new way of eating and a healthier lifestyle. One major motivator for most people is health. One major motivator is also the avoidance of adverse outcomes. Let health and weight loss be your reward. But when your rewards don't come soon enough, let avoidance be your motivation. Use the material in the following chapter as information, but also as motivation.

CHAPTER 2

THE DIET

SUMMARY

- The more you cut animal products out of your diet, the more weight you may be able to lose.
- The more you cut out junk food, the more weight you can lose.
- Eat natural, nutrient dense foods with names you can pronounce.
- Do your best to eliminate processed foods and chemicals.
- Make a vegan diet work for you by making it your own.

3 YOUR HEALTH AS DETERMINED BY YOUR MEASUREMENTS

I have lost 20 pounds by adopting a vegan diet. I feel great and have no cravings nor desires to return to my old habits.

<u>Why Take Your Measurements?</u>
Getting on the scale can be a major difficulty for some people. All kinds of feelings can come rushing in from dread to despair. But those bad feelings can change to feelings of joy and excitement as your health and physique improve. They say bad physical feelings are expressed in the body as the same chemicals that bad mental feelings are. When you feel better physically, you should therefore feel better mentally as well.

Knowing your starting points may make you feel bad at first, but watching your measurements improve can make you feel great. Researchers have determined certain specific measurements as either related to health or associated with disease. By knowing these predetermined numbers and using them as goals, you can help yourself objectively become healthier and avoid disease.

Have fun with them. Don't take yourself too seriously; just play along. They are not meant to make you feel bad or compare you to others as either superior or inferior. They are just measurements. Instead, use them as motivation. Soon, you'll be able to look back on them an see how far you have come.

Measuring Exercise #1: Predicting Your Risk of High Blood Pressure, Type 2 Diabetes, High cholesterol, and Heart Disease

Please:
- Get some string.
- Men cut a piece of string 40 inches long.
- Ladies cut a piece of string 35 inches long.
- Take your string and try to fit it around your waist.

I know this does not seem like a lot of string. You have to be pretty slim to make this length fit around your waist. Studies show though that having a waist circumference larger than this increases your risk of high blood pressure, type 2 diabetes, high cholesterol, and heart disease.[79]

Put this string away for now. This can be a long-term goal for you. Save that string, maybe by your scale, and try it again occasionally, for motivation.

We have heard that men having beer bellies (or women that have a bigger belly than hips) is harmful to your health. When the fat is deposited on your stomach, it goes under your skin, but it also goes in between and even in your internal organs. The new health crisis because of this is nonalcoholic fatty liver disease. Risk factors for this include obesity, gastric bypass surgery, high cholesterol, and type 2 diabetes. You may not have symptoms, or you might experience abdominal pain, fatigue, swelling in your belly, and yellow of your skin and eyes. As the disease progresses the liver begins to scar and stop functioning. This is cirrhosis and may include the symptoms of

---

[79] These numbers vary depending on your ethnic group. You can ask your doctor about a healthy waist measurement for you.

mental confusion, internal bleeding, and fluid retention.

Yes, we normally think of cirrhosis of the liver as being caused by excess alcohol. This is the same kind of thing and like alcoholic related cirrhosis, it can require a liver transplant.

Waist circumference is also related to high blood pressure. So many things are intricately related in our body. The good news though is if you do something good for one part of your body, you can often see health benefits in other parts of your body, too.

<u>Measuring Exercise #2: Your Waist Circumference</u>
Get a string or cloth measuring tape and measure your waist. Guys don't use your metal tape from construction. You need a soft measuring tape this time.

- Stand up.
- Start at your hips.
- Measure all the way around with the tape measure level with your belly button.
- Don't pull the tape measure tight and don't hold your breath.
- Record your measurement.

Write down the date: ___________________
And your measurement in inches here:
____

It is a good idea to keep this measurement an indicator early in your program. By repeating this measurement, you can track your progress. A lot of people do this with clothing. I know a lot of men do not like to weigh themselves, but when their pants don't fit or they must use a different notch on their belt, they know something has changed. You may also notice that sometimes when you seem to be stuck at a weight, your body composition may be changing. For instance, you could be gaining muscle. Since muscle weighs more than fat, you can lose fat while gaining muscle thus maintaining weight. However, you may see changes in your waist circumference or other body measurements.

<u>Measuring Exercise #3: Sagittal Abdominal Height</u>
You are probably going to need a buddy to help you with this one.

You are going to need:

- a ruler
- either a yardstick or something else long and straight.

Lay on your back on a hard surface. You don't want to be on a bed or other surface that you sink into for this one.

With your knees bent and feet flat on the floor, place your yardstick across your stomach at about the level of your belly button or whatever spot is narrowest. Take your ruler and measure from the floor to the height of the yardstick coming across your abdomen, like this:

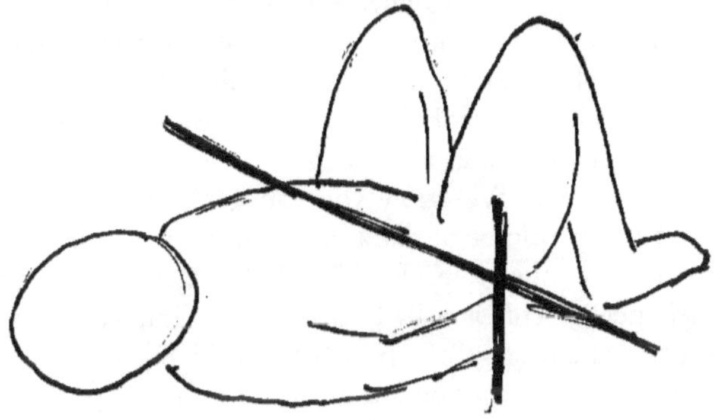

Try to have the yardstick cross just above the top of your hip. This is called your sagittal or supine abdominal height (SAH). Let's call it our stomach height.

Write down your stomach height here: _______________
Write down the date here: _______________

Am I at risk for heart disease, insulin resistance, and Alzheimer's? (I'll tell how to fill this out in the section "Why do these Measurements Matter?" in just a bit.) ______________ yes ______________ no

Now don't feel bad if this height seems excessive. I doubt this is something that anyone has ever asked you to do. I'm fairly certain that no one has ever told you this was important.

We accumulate fat in our bodies in different places. I am sure you have heard that women get fat on their hips and rear ends, and that men get fat on their stomachs. But the problem with this fat is not how it looks, as much as what it does to your internal organs. The more fat you have on your midsection, the more it starts to work its way between your organs. The fat underneath your skin isn't so bad. The fat between your organs is. The larger your stomach height, the more likely you are to have excessive fat between your organs and even inside of them. This internal organ fat in the liver we mentioned already as nonalcoholic fatty liver disease. Incidentally, nonalcoholic fatty liver disease is associated with intakes of soft drinks and meats.[80]

Now, men. We know you can get a beer belly, which in itself is a predictor of disease. But when you run out of room for fat on your stomach, men tend to get rolls of fat behind their necks. This is a bad sign. This accumulation of fat may happen at any stage of a beer belly, and while it may be genetic, it may also be that you ate the same foods as your other male relatives who may very well be at risk for disease, too.

Take your cell phone and snap a selfie of the back of your neck and the side of you neck.

---

[80] ShiraZelber-Sagi, DoritNitzan-Kaluski, Rebecca Goldsmith, Muriel Webb, Laurie Blendis, Zamir Halpern, Ran Oren. Long term nutritional intake and the risk for non-alcoholic fatty liver disease (NAFLD): A population based study. Journal of Hepatology. Volume 47, Issue 5, November 2007, Pages 711-717.

Do you have any sign of rolls?
I have rolls of fat on the back of my neck.
_______ yes or _________no
Today's date is: ___________________

If you have rolls of fat on the back of your neck, use these pictures as your motivation. If you feel the urge to be gluttonous, get out your phone and give yourself a gentle reminder.

<u>Measuring Exercise #4: Neck Circumference</u>
You will need a long piece of string (or ribbon) and a measuring tape or yard stick.

Take your string and put it around your neck at the middle of your neck. You may want to use a ribbon instead if the skin on your neck is delicate. Hold the points of the string where they meet and then measure the length of your string with your yard stick or measuring tape. I suggest using a string or ribbon because putting the measuring tape directly against your neck can be uncomfortable, number one, but also, we all tend to cheat a little when we use a measuring tape. Who among us has not sucked in their gut when measuring their waist? Measuring your gut is one thing, but measuring your neck is a very important measurement of your health and we want it to be accurate with no built-in self-denial.

Write down your measurement for neck circumference here: ___________ inches.

If you are a man, is your neck circumference greater than 17 inches? _____________yes or _____________no

If you are a woman, is your neck circumference greater than 16 inches? _____________yes or ______no

If your neck circumference is greater than these measurements, you can be at greater risk for sleep apnea and its associated conditions such as high blood pressure.

Might my neck circumference put me at greater risk of various health conditions? (See "Why do these Measurements Matter?" next.)

___________yes or ___________no

<u>Why do these Measurements Matter?</u>
- Your stomach height is a strong predictor of heart disease.
- For both men and women, your stomach height should be less than 9.8 inches (about nine and three quarters).
- If you have a stomach height over 9.8 inches, you are at risk of Alzheimer's disease and even a lower than normal brain volume.
- If you have a stomach height of over 12 inches, you also are at risk for cardiovascular disease and insulin resistance (a precursor to diabetes).
- If you have a neck circumference greater than 17 inches for men or 16 inches for women, you are at a greater risk of sleep apnea and its related problems of high blood pressure, heart attack, and stroke.

Now go back and check the blank "yes" or "no" above where it asks you if you are at risk for heart disease, insulin resistance, and Alzheimer's. Mark "yes" if you stomach height is over 9.8 inches (about 9 ¾"). If your stomach height is over 12 inches, mark it again and put a star or something that will make you notice it. If your neck circumference is over 17 inches (men) or 16 inches (women) mark "yes" in for the last question above. Start talking about these numbers. People don't know about them. Get your friends to lie down and measure their stomach height. You may be the one who puts them on the path to health instead of a life looking forward to heart disease, diabetes, stroke, and Alzheimer's.

You can change these numbers! But if you don't know you

are at risk, you can't do anything to change them. Use these numbers to motivate you in your decision to go vegan.

<u>How to Weigh Yourself.</u>

You know what is coming next. You're right. I'm going to ask you to measure your weight.

Now there is a reason why I have not asked you to do this yet, and that is because I, number one, think that you are more than a number. You are a wonderful, worthwhile person, and you were put here for a reason. And if you haven't found that reason yet, I know you will, because everyone has a reason for being here, or we wouldn't be here in the first place.

The second reason is because I wanted you to start thinking about yourself, your body, and your weight in terms of your health and not just a number. Numbers change and people change. We can all become better, regardless of what the scale (or any other number) tells us. The judge of our value is not a number on the scale.

So, yes, I want you to weight yourself. In fact, I want you to weight yourself every day from here on out, or at least while you are reading this book. Be sure to weigh yourself frequently though as we know that weighing yourself less than once a week is associated with weight gain and obesity. But before you go hop on the scale let's cover a few things first.

First, you need a good scale. It should be relatively new and digital. If you have an old bathroom scale that has been banged around, stored on its side, the kids have jumped on, or any such thing that may make it inaccurate, I wouldn't bother with it. You also want to try to use the same scale all the time. If you weight yourself at the gym, and the scale is not balanced, it will not give you an accurate weight. Most of the scales at gyms are the kind of scales you see at a doctor's office. These are called a weight beam scale. They have two bars each with weights on them. If you push these weights all the way to the left the beam should be perfectly level and be floating on the right. If when you push these weights all the way to the left, the bar on the right is not level with the floor, that is, either goes up or down, the scale is out of balance and must be adjusted with the screws on the left of the bars so that the beam is perfectly leveled and therefore "zeroed." That is, if it is not zeroed it thinks that either something is already on the scale or it subtracts something from your weight. Having the beam balanced means that the scale knows that nothing is being weighed and the measurement is thus zero. If you try to take your weight on a scale that is not zeroed, you will never have an exact weight. The other thing that people commonly do on these scales is not moving the weights on the beams properly. When you slide the larger of the weights, you must be sure that the weights settle into the little nooks directly under the numbers, or again, your measurement will not be accurate.

If you have a digital scale, you must make sure that it will weigh you. If you are very heavy, you want to make sure that you know how much you weigh so that you can see how much you lose. You should also try, at least once, to put an object of know weight on your scale and see that it measures it accurately. You might have a dumbbell or other weight that you can put on the scale and measure. You could also hold the weight with you on the scale and make sure that it adds the appropriate amount. If your scale does not read appropriately, look at your scale directions and see if you can adjust it in some way. The other thing to consider is to make sure that you can see the numbers on the scale when you are on it. If you have to lean forward or to the side to try to see your weight, look for a different scale. They make digital scales with the readout on a small screen attached to the scale with a wire for this purpose. Unfortunately, these scales can be very expensive. You may have to enlist the help your spouse or a friend if you can't see your weight on your scale. You might even have a local doctor or chiropractor who will let you pop in and take your weight on a regular basis. (My husband is a chiropractor and they are very much into health and wellness including nutrition.)

I used to use an old bathroom scale. Before I got on the scale, I would make sure that it read zero. If it didn't, I would adjust the dial, so it did. I thought I was doing a good thing, but then I went to the gym and weighted myself. Well, my weight was not the same. Yes, it was probably higher. And, yes, I would get discouraged. So, I would just blame the lousy scale at the YMCA and everyone beating up on it. Then I went to the doctor's office. Yes, again it was more. I knew better than to complain but could there really be a ten- or fifteen-pound difference between my trusty bathroom scale and the doctor's office. Again, you guessed it, I blamed the doctor's office. Those lousy nurses. They didn't zero their scale. Here I was losing weight. I had to be losing weight. My numbers on my scale were going down. Yes, I was losing weight, but I really had no idea how much because of my beat-up, old spring-scale.

So, do yourself a favor, and get yourself a good digital scale if you don't have one. A scale is a good tool to help you have fun motivating yourself as your numbers drop.

When to Weigh Yourself.

The best time to weigh yourself is first thing in the morning after you have gone to the bathroom. For the most accurate results, weight yourself in the nude. You can make this a daily habit by keeping your scale in the bathroom and weighing yourself as you wait for the shower to warm up. This gives you a set time, when you should be at your lightest to weigh yourself. Please do not get in the habit of weighing yourself with clothing or shoes on. These can all add pounds to your weight. Plus, you change your clothes daily with the weather and with the season, so it is just more accurate to weigh yourself naked.

You should keep track of your weight, but I can understand why you may not want to. Yes, it can be discouraging sometimes, but it can be highly motivating, too. By weighing yourself you have an easy way of monitoring yourself, and what gets monitored can be changed.

<u>Measuring Exercise: Your Weight</u>
If it is not first thing in the morning, wait until tomorrow.
If it is, please weight yourself now.

My weight: _______________________________
Date:_________________________________

<u>How Often to Weigh Yourself?</u>
I recommend weighing yourself daily. Why? First, your weight really does change daily, which I will go into in a minute. Secondly, if you weigh yourself weekly or any less than that, it really does not give you the opportunity to make corrections quickly. Everyone is different. One weight loss tip may work for someone else, but not for you. If you wait two weeks or a month to check your weight, this can result in a lot of pounds and a lot of discouragement if this tip is not working for you.

Now I know a lot of people are going to be up in arms that I say you should weight yourself daily. Certainly, there are a lot of things that can account for daily variations. Daily weighing, however, establishes a good habit: Get up, use the bathroom, weight yourself naked while the shower is warming up, or whatever your routine. The idea is that you get in an easy to follow habit. It is a lot harder to think of weighting yourself say Sunday morning at 8:00 p.m. or Monday morning at six than it is to remember to do it daily as you get in the shower, etc. Also remember: Anything less that one weekly weighing is related to weight gain.

<u>What can Change your Weight on a Daily Basis?</u>
Weight change on daily basis is normal. This may be due to fat loss, muscle gain, inflammation, and water retention.

Certainly, the scale should show an overall trend toward a healthy weight when we are eating appropriately, being physically active, and healthy. Our goal though is a reduction in body fat. If we exercise a lot or start a completely new weightlifting program though we may see an overall weight gain due to muscle increases if body fat stays constant. Muscle weights more than fat, so you could conceivably weight more due to muscle gain if fat is not lost. (This is why it is good to take some body measurements other than weight also.)

Water retention can also add to your weight. Ironically, it you don't drink enough water, your body wants to hold onto it more. You need water for the body's metabolic processes and if you don't drink enough water, toxins, including all the normal by-products of metabolism, won't get flushed from your system. We know that premenstrual syndrome can cause weight gain due to water retention, so be sure to drink to thirst. You probably want to drink more in fact because thirst tends to be a later sign of dehydration. Women before their periods also tend to crave so-called comfort foods, foods high in carbohydrates. So, don't blame it on water-weight if you know you have been overdoing it!

Eating too much salt can also make it appear as if you have gained weight. The more salt (sodium) you eat, the more it will pull fluids into your cells. This can show as an overall gain in weight if you have a high sodium diet most days, or as a gain in weight if you ate a lot of salt on any given day. Retaining too much water due to excessive salt is not a good thing. This overall inflammation of the body is linked to disease including heart disease and cancer. Eating salty foods may also cause you to eat more than you would otherwise. Salt is one of those pleasure triggers for many people that cause us to eat more than we should. Just think, "Would I eat more plain popcorn or more movie-theater salty popcorn even without their 'butter?'" If you're like me, no doubt the movie theater kind. You physically have to take it away and goodness knows how much soda you'll want to drink with it!

Another cause for daily weight fluctuations is the loss of glycogen from the muscles. Glycogen is the body's method for storing quick energy for bursts of energy. Thus, it is stored close to where it is used, that is, the muscles, as well as the liver. The more you do aerobic exercise with anaerobic bursts, the more glycogen you will build. That is, if you do high-intensity bursts of exercise in which the muscles have little time to get oxygen, you use more glycogen and you will build more glycogen in the days after exercise. You probably have heard this if you ever have taken a spinning (stationary cycling) class. Glycogen holds a lot of water, so if you use it a lot you may notice weight gain the following day. Weight gain after exercise may also be due to inflammation (not so good), as well. However, if you do not eat many carbohydrates after a hard bout of exercise, you will not build glycogen and may show some weight loss. This then is detrimental as you will not build glycogen and not be able to perform as well during anaerobic exercise (exercise without time enough to get air, e.g. sprints). In fact, extreme care should be used when trying to do anaerobic sprinting exercises during a ketogenic diet. You may wind-up on the floor passing out instead of having a great high-energy class.

Remember too that each meal you eat has its own weight. Therefore I recommend weighing yourself at the same time of day (after you use the bathroom in the morning). Everything you eat has weight and certain foods will make you want to drink more fluids and retain more water in your body and your digestive tract. A pint is a pound the world around. That's right. Two cups of water weights one pound.

Keeping track of your weight can keep you motivated. But remember again, you are more than a number. Keep in mind the trend in your weight. A week of numbers going generally down (toward a healthy weight) is great, but more than a couple days of your weight going up can be cause for concern. Think back to what might be going on. Are you dehydrated and should be drinking more water? Did you eat too much salt? Ladies, are you going to get your period soon? Did you exercise hard? Did you eat a big, heavy meal that is still in your system? Or, have you simply been eating too much of the wrong foods lately?

<u>So How Much Should You Weight?</u>
This is a very good question and surprisingly it is a very

complicated one. Insurance companies, not doctors, have historically taken the lead in the development of height and weight tables. They want to see which of their clients will live the longest and the shortest amounts of time so that they can charge them accordingly. Why not give someone a good price if you know that you can get payments out of them for a very long time? And, why should they give someone a good price if they know they might keel over in the next couple of years? Originally, tables showed average weights for the insured. These showed that weights increased with age. In the time of their development, pneumonia and tuberculosis were major killers and this extra weight gain was considered healthy to help fend off disease and to be used in times of illness. Being underweight compared to the rest of the population was considered undesirable and unhealthy. As infectious disease was contained, new height and weight tables emerged as the causes of mortality changed. Insurance company tables are not necessarily ideal weights, but they are those associated with the lowest mortality (death).[81] Weight gain with age is known as a factor in disease.

The calculation of body mass index is now the norm because it is known to be associated with overall mortality. In all age groups, those with the highest body mass index have the highest risk of death. This holds true for all causes, cardiovascular disease, cancer, and other diseases and the rates of risk increase as weight increases.[82]

To find your BMI, multiply your weight in pounds by 703 and divide the result by your height in inches squared. That is, weight (lbs.) X 703 / height^2 (in). This is also equal to weight (kg) / height^2 (m). You can find free BMI calculators online.

---

[81] Weigley ES. Average? Ideal? Desirable? A brief overview of height-weight tables in the United States. Journal of the American Dietetic Association [01 Apr 1984, 84(4):417-423].

[82] Eugenia E. Calle, Ph.D., Michael J. Thun, M.D., Jennifer M. Petrelli, M.P.H., Carmen Rodriguez, M.D., M.P.H., and Clark W. Heath, Jr., M.D. Body-Mass Index and Mortality in a Prospective Cohort of U.S. Adults. N Engl J Med 1999; 341:1097-1105

Alternately, you could use the following table[83] in which you can either use you measurements in the metric system or English system to find your BMI and its meaning:

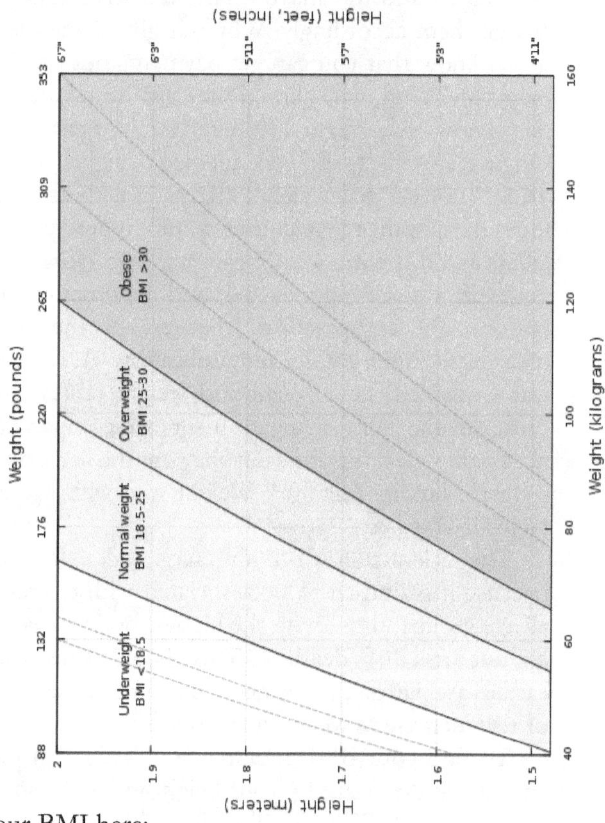

Record your BMI here: _________________
Date:________________
You can check this on occasion as well.

____

[83] Amfucia using gnuplot and inkscape. BMI chart, intended as an improvement for the one currently on the English Wikipedia page. Curved lines show the principle cutoffs between the various BMI categories, as specified by the WH. Sept 21, 2017.
https://commons.wikimedia.org/wiki/File:BMI_chart.svg

The following graphic developed by the Centers for Disease Control and Prevention (CDC), United States Department of Health and Human Services (HHS) might be an easier way to look things up. The information is not delivered in a very tactful way (using a belt), but it does get the information across. Figure you should weigh less than these numbers.[84]

---

[84] Obesity table. Adult Obesity-CDC Vital Signs-August 2010.pdf. Centers for Disease Control and Prevention, part of the United States Department of Health and Human Services. 21 August 2012.

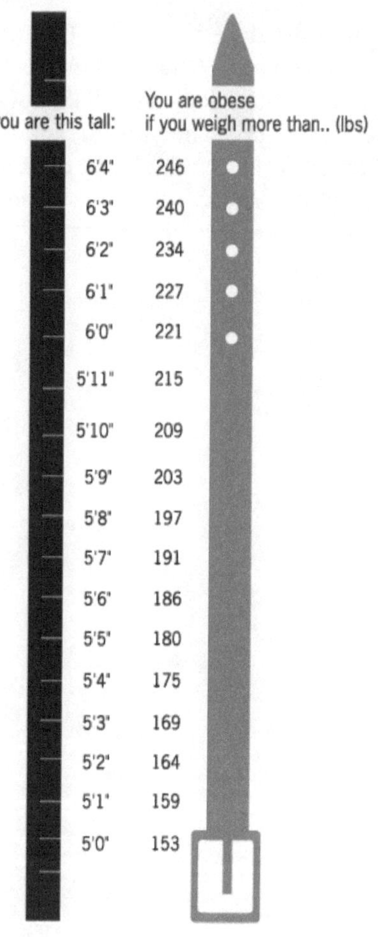

Obesity Table: You are obese if you are this tall, and weigh more than: 6'4" – 246lbs. 6'3" – 240lbs. 6'2" – 234lbs. 6'1" – 227lbs. 6'0" – 221lbs. 5'11" – 215lbs. 5'10" – 209lbs. 5'9" – 203lbs. 5'8" – 197lbs. 5'7" – 191lbs. 5'6" – 186lbs. 5'5" – 180lbs. 5'4" – 175lbs. 5'3" – 169lbs. 5'2" – 164lbs. 5'1" – 159lbs. 5'0" – 153lbs.

These numbers are rather abstract for most people. Thus, it is still useful to look at the good, old-fashioned Met Life Insurance tables to see your actual weight. Afterall, we are still people who think in terms of weight and not a single digit, strange number that somehow relates to it. It is also hard to think in terms of BMI percentiles which you might sometimes see. When was the last time someone asked you your BMI after all? We are not used to thinking that way. If you have ever bought life insurance, you will know that these are the tables that they use and your insurance salesman will quote you a rate that is based on where you fit in these tables and your other insurance risks. Just for the record, those high-risk behaviors that may cause you to receive a more expensive quote, or be denied insurance altogether, include smoking cigarettes or cigars, chewing tobacco, skydiving, being in a high risk profession such as underwater welding, underground mining, or firefighting, scuba diving, car racing, and problems with your medical history.

Most of us might just be more comfortable looking at the Metropolitan Height and Weight Tables for Men and Women. Don't worry so much about frame size. There are ways to calculates it, but you should have a general idea of how you compare to others by the width/size of your bones in your wrist and shoulders.

Ideal Weight Chart for Men:

Height	Small Frame	Med. Frame	Large Frame
6'4"	162 - 176 lb	171 - 187 lb	181 - 207 lb
6'3"	158 - 172 lb	167 - 182 lb	176 - 202 lb
6'2"	155 - 168 lb	164 - 178 lb	172 - 197 lb
6'1"	152 - 164 lb	160 - 174 lb	168 - 192 lb
6'	149 - 160 lb	157 - 170 lb	164 - 188 lb
5'11"	146 - 157 lb	154 - 166 lb	161 - 184 lb
5'10"	144 - 154 lb	151 - 163 lb	158 - 180 lb
5'9"	142 - 151 lb	148 - 160 lb	155 - 176 lb
5'8"	140 - 148 lb	145 - 157 lb	152 - 172 lb
5'7"	138 - 145 lb	142 - 154 lb	149 - 168 lb
5'6"	136 - 142 lb	139 - 151 lb	146 - 164 lb
5'5"	134 - 140 lb	137 - 148 lb	144 - 160 lb
5'4"	132 - 138 lb	135 - 145 lb	142 - 156 lb
5'3"	130 - 136 lb	133 - 143 lb	140 - 153 lb
5'2"	128 - 134 lb	131 - 141 lb	138 - 150 lb

From height and weight tables of the Metropolitan Life Insurance Company, 1983. The ideal weight given in these tables are for ages 25 to 59. The ideal weight assumes you are wearing shoes with 1-inch heels and indoor clothing weighing 5 pounds.

Ideal Weight Chart for Women:

Height	Small Frame	Med. Frame	Large Frame
6'	138-151 lb	148-162 lb	158-179 lb
5'11"	135-148 lb	145-159 lb	155-176 lb
5'10"	132-145 lb	142-156 lb	152-173 lb
5'9"	129-142 lb	139-153 lb	149-170 lb
5'8"	126-139 lb	136-150 lb	146-167 lb
5'7"	123-136 lb	133-147 lb	143-163 lb
5'6"	120-133 lb	130-144 lb	140-159 lb
5'5"	117-130 lb	127-141 lb	137-155 lb
5'4"	114-127 lb	124-138 lb	134-151 lb
5'3"	111-124 lb	121-135 lb	131-147 lb
5'2"	108-121 lb	118-132 lb	128-143 lb
5'1"	106–118 lb	115-129 lb	125-140 lb
5'	104-115 lb	113-126 lb	122-137 lb
4'11"	103-113 lb	111-123 lb	120-134 lb
4'10"	102-111 lb	109-121 lb	118-131 lb

From height and weight tables of the Metropolitan Life Insurance Company, 1983. The ideal weight given in these tables are for ages 25 to 59. The ideal weight assumes you are wearing shoes with 1-inch heels and indoor clothing weighing 5 pounds.

Make a note of how you fit in these tables here for reference if you like along with the date:

____

CHAPTER 3

YOUR HEALTH AS DETERMINED BY YOUR MEASUREMENTS

SUMMARY

- Taking your measurements is not meant to make you feel bad. Use it as motivation and to help determine your risk of disease.
- Take your measurements to keep track of your progress and make any corrections to your diet and life-style before things get out of hand.

4 RECLAIMING YOUR HEALTH PHYSICALLY & MENTALLY

I've lost 20 pounds since becoming a near-vegan. My cholesterol has fallen from 230 to 160. I've kept it off for nearly 3 years now.

<u>The Action Plan for Getting Anything Accomplished.</u>
The first step in solving any problem is realizing you have a problem. I think you have established that. If you need some more motivation make sure that you do the various measuring exercises and mental, visualization activities in this book. The second step is finding solutions that work. By continuing to read about the experiences of the individuals in this book, you can see that this approach has worked for others and may very well work for you, too. The third step is having motivation to continue. Motivating yourself will keep you going. We all have bad days and good days, too. Read the visualization exercises here in to keep you motivated. If you need more motivation, try looking into the many other various reasons for becoming a vegetarian. People that become vegetarian with a devout belief that it is wrong to kill stay devoted to vegetarianism for themselves and their animal friends as well. Research health, religion, environment, animal rights, and philosophy to find a reason besides yourself to keep you vegetarian. Wanting a taste

of something means very little to you if you believe it is immoral. Find a reason outside of yourself to keep your motivated to stay vegetarian for your health. The final step in resilience[85] is finding a support system. Anyone who has a problem and finds others that they can talk to that had a similar problem and solved it will be a great help. There are many vegetarian/vegan social groups out there. There are many ways of connecting over the internet. There are stories of many people in Chapter 7 that you can read and reread to give you inspiration. I always try to tell new vegetarians to find a vegetarian potluck in their area to attend. Potlucks enable you to connect with new people while sampling a wide variety of dishes. This way you can learn from people's experiences, plus find out about new foods and cooking techniques by trying a bite rather than trying to figure everything out on your own.

<u>What Are You Dying For?</u>

The following are all health outcomes to which excessive weight is a risk factor. I would like to go over in some detail each of these conditions, first, to inform you, and second, to, quite frankly, scare you. As I go over each of these conditions, I would like you to visualize in great detail what each of these diagnoses would mean to you and your family. Think how they would feel physically. Think of how they would feel mentally. Think of what they would do to your family. What would they do to you financially? Would you be able to work? How would they change your daily life? What if you died? What would happen to your family?

I know it is horrible to think of these things. But, hopefully, if you really picture what life would be like if you continue the path that you are on, you can change things, before it is too late.

If you have a loved one who had these problems, or perhaps even died from one of these conditions, I thoroughly understand if you want to skip reading a certain section. I think

---

[85] This is part of my doctorate work.

about my father who died from botched surgery for stage-one esophageal cancer. I have played repeatedly in my mind what happened to him. I have felt such emotion every time I have thought of it. I can bring myself to tears every time if I think about it enough. Some may say that is not healthy, but I know that I will never ever follow in his path nor do some of the things he did (e.g. drink scalding-hot drinks). I never ever want my children to endure such a level of grief. We all must go sometime, but I would rather go peacefully in my own bed than go out with horrible, dramatic suffering whether it be short or long.

My mom once told me, "You do what you can, and then the rest is just a roll of the dice."

You know what? I absolutely do not believe that!

There are so many things that we can do right now to be healthier and happier, so let's make this day a new beginning. You are smarter than you were yesterday, and you can be healthier than you were yesterday, too.

I always tell the kids: "Sometimes knowing what you don't want to do is just as important as knowing what you want to do."

So, indulge me. Let's condition our brains for the better.

<u>Known Outcomes of Excess Weight.</u>

There are many known outcomes to carrying excess weight. Some relate to physical health. Some relate to your mental health. Some relate to your social health.

Right now, we are going to focus on your physical health.

I am extremely serious about this next part. I want you to put this book down, stop everything else you are doing, and call your physician right now if you experience any of these symptoms:

- Pain in your chest, neck, or jaw
- Pressure or squeezing in your chest
- Shortness of breath at rest or relaxation
- Dizziness
- Fainting

- Swollen ankles (edema)
- Difficulty breathing when you are lying down
- Shortness of breath or coughing when lying down or sleeping
- Feeling like you are having rapid, hard, or abnormal heart beats
- Feeling like you are having irregular heart beats
- Aching, crampy, tired, or burning pain in the legs
- Unusual shortness of breath or fatigue while doing your normal activities

These are all major signs and symptoms of disease and need to be addressed by you physician. If you are experiencing any of these, you need to call your doctor. And I will emphasize, you should not do any type of exercise program if you are experiencing any of these. You need to be evaluated by your doctor. Also, if you smoke, you are at high risk for health problems and should be evaluated by a physician.

I repeat this information from the beginning of the book to make sure that you have the information to make sure you take care of yourself. These can be signs of coronary artery disease, hypertension, problems with glucose metabolism, high cholesterol levels, and other problems. If you experience any of these, or any other worrisome signs or symptoms, call you doctor and get it checked out. It is always better to be safe than sorry.

Here is how the CDC illustrates their research on the know medical complications of obesity (notice their graphics illustrates a relatively slim obese person):

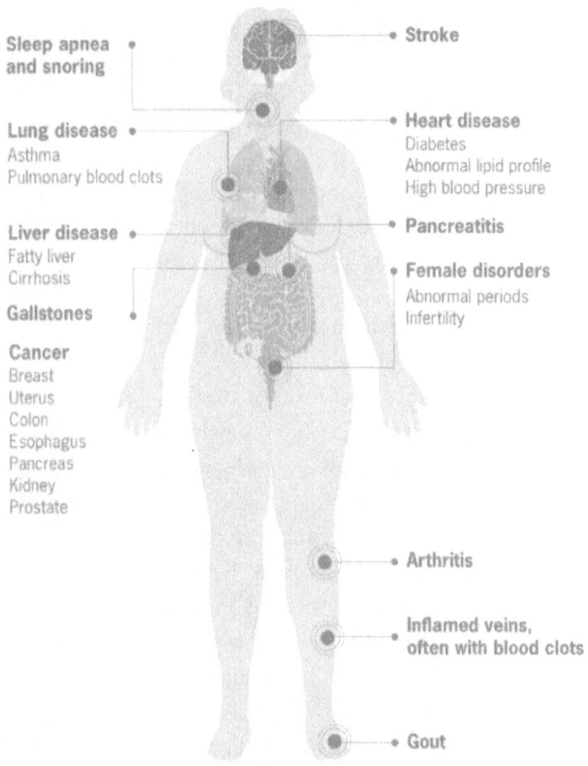

Medical Complications of Obesity – Obesity affects many body parts: brain (stroke); throat (sleep apnea, snoring); lungs (lung disease, asthma, pulmonary blood clots); heart (heart disease, diabetes, abnormal lipid profile, high blood pressure); liver (liver disease, fatty liver, cirrhosis); pancreas (pancreatitis); gall bladder (gallstones); uterus (female disorders, abnormal periods, infertility); knees (arthritis); calves (inflamed veins, often with blood clots); feet (gout); breast, uterus, colon, esophagus, pancreas, kidney, prostate (cancer).[86]

---

[86] CDC Vital Signs. Aug 2010. Medical Complications of Obesity. Adapted from Yale University Rudd Center for Food Policy and Obesity. https://www.cdc.gov/vitalsigns/adultobesity/infographic.html

<u>Mental Conditioning Exercises for Health and Longevity.</u>
This next section is part of your mental conditioning for becoming a healthier, slimmer person. This section is meant to help motivate you. If any section is too much to do or think about, skip it.

When you want to have something that you know really isn't good for you, the following feelings and emotions that you may experience are the kinds of things that can help keep you motivated.

For each of these mental exercises, you can:

- Read them to yourself;
- Think deeply about them as you read;
- Close your eyes after you read and really try to experience and feel through your imagination what each might be like;
- You could also have someone else, like a friend, spouse, or therapist read them to while you and visualize them as they read;
- The more you allow yourself to feel , the more you will internalize the results;
- The basic format will be: Think, feel, then smash! That is, think about the information and allow yourself to feel what your future might be like if these bad events come about, then smash that image so that it is gone forever. You can do this in any way that you want to visualize. You could smash the bad image on the ground, break it with and hammer, blow it up and see it pop, or even make flowers grow out of it destroying the bad image of illness and disease and replacing it with a new image of health, happiness, love, and longevity. The point is to feel the bad results and then decide at your very core that this bad image is not what your future life will

be. Have fun and make it as real as you want. Replace the bad with a new good image. You can use this psychological technique as a motivational tool in any area of your life including your diet.

<u>Mental Conditioning Exercise: Visualizing Your Body.</u>
Use the information you now have for motivation, not discouragement. Today is a new day.

Close your eyes. Think about your body. Think about measuring your body. Does the simple act of measuring your body make you feel bad? Think about the measurement of your stomach while lying on your back. Was it uncomfortable to do? Was it uncomfortable to measure and think of the number?

Now, think about what that number means? Could you have heart disease in the future? Could you have heart disease now? What about insulin resistance that can lead to diabetes? What about Alzheimer's? Do these things worry you or do they darn right terrify you? Think about the back of your neck? Do you like how it looks or do you wish you never took those selfies?

Think long and hard about those things and then:

Write one thing down right now that you can do for your diet and your health:

____

____

When you think of this one thing, visualize what might happen to you if you don't keep this promise to yourself. Make it so real, that the thought of doing this thing is so repulsive to you that you would never dream of breaking this promise to yourself.

I am sure you came up with a great idea you can stick to. But in case you had a hard time, here are some ideas:

- Eat a green vegetable every day.
- Drink a big glass of water before eating.
- Trim any visible fat off any animal product you eat.
- Make Friday's a meat-free day. Try to make it completely vegetarian.

Mental Conditioning: Understanding the Consequences of High Blood Pressure.

Read and feel the following. The more you can experience it as real, the more you can work with zeal to not let this be you.

You've been feeling lightheaded and dizzy lately. You don't feel like you can do the things you used to. Sometimes you get a pounding in your head and sometimes you get a pounding in your chest. Your extra weight has increased the workload on your heart since it has to pump blood to a larger area. This extra pressure means more pressure on the artery wall and an increased heart rate. You've noticed these symptoms and it is time for a doctor's visit.

But even if you haven't noticed anything, this high blood pressure can be damaging your arteries. They are getting hard and narrow. This makes it more likely for you to have a heart attack or even a stroke.

What would you do then? What would happen to your family? How would they take care of you? You are supposed to be taking care of them. What would you do for money? How would you pay your bills?

This extra workload is making your heart grow bigger. There is more demand for oxygen and your heart is less able to maintain blood flow. You feel weak and tired. You can't do your normal activities.

This high blood pressure is damaging your kidneys.

It can damage your eyes. If you have diabetes, it can cause the small capillaries in the retina of your eye to bleed. It may even cause you to become blind, and what would happen then?

Now that you have this image in your head… Smash it! This will not be you! It won't be you anymore! Visualize getting rid of it however you want. Dissolve it! Smash it! Feel that it is real! This will NOT be you!

Now take a minute to think and compose yourself.

This does not have to be you. Right now, consider what you can do to keep the effects of high blood pressure out of your life. Then consider the following:

<u>Ten Things Your Can Do to Keep Hypertension Out of Your Life.</u>[87]
1. Lose extra pounds and watch your waistline
2. Exercise regularly
3. Eat a healthy diet
4. Reduce sodium in your diet
5. Limit the amount of alcohol you drink
6. Quit smoking
7. Cut back on caffeine
8. Reduce your stress
9. Monitor your blood pressure at home and see your doctor regularly
10. Get support

If you haven't noticed by now. Health is about many more things than just being a healthy weight. What is the sense in taking up smoking cigarettes for weight loss? Right? I am a nutritionist who is interested in whole-body health. Pick one of these items from the list above that you think you could do right now and circle it.

Next, write down here, one way you are going to make this happen:____

____

<u>Mental Exercise: Diabetes, Assessment and Prevention.</u>
Let's take a look at Type II Adult Onset Diabetes.
Again, read and think or have a friend read to you.

You are tired. Not just tired, you get exhausted. And you can't seem

---

[87] From "10 ways to control high blood pressure without medication." https://www.mayoclinic.org/diseases-conditions/high-blood-pressure/in-depth/high-blood-pressure/art-20046974

to control your hunger. High blood sugar is making you hungry and thirsty. Very thirsty. You're drinking all the time, but you are still hungry. And you are going to the bathroom all the time. You may be heavy, but you may have had a sudden, unexplained weight loss. The energy from your food is not getting to your cells. Even a moderate level of obesity dramatically increases your risk of diabetes. Insulin normally regulates blood sugar and yours isn't working. (If your experiencing anything like this, please stop now and call your doctor. If not, read on and visualize.)

This high blood sugar is causing numbness in your legs, burning in your feet, and tingling in the hands. This is caused by diabetic neuropathy and is from your years of high blood sugar levels. It hurts to walk. These high blood sugar levels mean you could have a heart attack or a stroke. Your kidneys could shut down. You could have to go on medications, or worse, dialysis. Your vision is being damaged. You might even go blind.

Your skin is not the same. You get sores and infections that don't seem to heal. Your blood pressure is high, and we know all the complications that can cause. All this and you have to take medications or injections multiple times a day and you have to keep track of everything you eat. Your kids or grandkids ask you about the shots and it has gotten difficult to eat anywhere but at home.

There must be a better way. Medications won't solve this problem. Diet and weight loss can treat it. In fact, they can reverse it. Better yet, let's reverse it altogether! Picture this tired, sore person. This will not be you! Take this person and hit her over the head with a head of lettuce! Visualize her disappearing. Chase her out of here. She will not be you. Say, "I will not be controlled by my lust for food. I will take control!"

Now write one thing that you will do to keep diabetes out of your life:____

<u>Mental Exercise: Atherosclerosis, Heart Disease, Stroke.</u>
Once again, let's use the power of the carrot and the stick to get up our motivation. This time let us consider the effects of atherosclerosis and heart disease. Let's do thing differently this time. Let's learn about symptoms first and save our visualization to the end.

If you are like most of us, you know of someone or even lost a family member who has had heart disease. You seem to be on the road to it now, too. Atherosclerosis, hardening of the arteries, is ten times more prevalent in those who are obese. The fatty deposits build up in arteries that supply the heart. The narrowed arteries and reduced blood flow to your heart may be causing chest pain called angina, and if it becomes worse it could even be a heart attack where part of the heart starts to die because blood flow to the heart itself is blocked. If you develop a blood clot and it happens to get stuck in one of the narrowed arteries leading to the brain, you can have a stroke. And what would you do then? Would you even be able to do anything? Or would you wind-up in a rehab facility, a financial and psychological burden on your family?

If your developing narrowing of the arteries, you can't supply enough oxygen-rich blood to your heart. This is especially bad when the heart is beating hard during exercise. You may not be noticing it yet, but as the disease progresses, you'll begin to develop symptoms.

Angina is chest pain. Not just pain, pain like someone standing on your chest. They describe it as pressure or tightness in the middle or left side of the chest. It can be triggered by physical effort or emotional stress. If you're lucky, it can go away within minutes, or it can last. It can also be experienced as a fast, sharp pain in the neck, arm or back. This is especially true in women.

You may also develop shortness of breath. Since your heart can't pump enough blood to get the oxygen to your cells, you can have shortness of breath. This can cause extreme fatigue and make it difficult to do most anything.

Should your arteries become completely blocked, you will have a heart attack. This feels like your chest is being crushed by pressure accompanied by pain in your shoulder or arm, and often shortness of breath and sweating. As a woman, you may have neck or jaw pain, arm pain, back pain, or stomach pain, and the symptoms may be less specific and severe, but no less dangerous or deadly. Symptoms may last or leave and then come back.

Women are somewhat more likely than men are to experience less typical signs and symptoms of a heart attack, such as neck or jaw pain. Sometimes a heart attack occurs without any apparent signs or symptoms. You might break out in a cold sweat, have nausea or lightheadedness. If you are having any of these symptoms, you know you should get medical assistance.

Not everyone gets the typical symptoms, but if you ever have these signs that are new or unusual to you, are severe, or several are present, you need to call 911.

The American Stroke Association uses the pneumonic "FAST" to help people remember the signs. Signs of a stroke from the American Stroke Association include:

"F.A.S.T.:
- Face Drooping:
  Does one side of the face droop or is it numb? Ask the person to smile. Is the person's smile uneven or lopsided?
- Arm Weakness:
  Is one arm weak or numb? Ask the person to raise both arms. Does one arm drift downward?
- Speech Difficulty:
  Is speech slurred? Is the person unable to speak or hard to understand? Ask the person to repeat a simple sentence.
- Time to call 911: If the person shows any of these symptoms, even if the symptoms go away, call 9-1-1 and get them to the hospital immediately."[88]

And other symptoms may occur that also need attention:
- "Sudden NUMBNESS or weakness of face, arm, or leg, especially on one side of the body.

---

[88]Stroke Symptoms, American Stroke Association.
https://www.strokeassociation.org/en/about-stroke/stroke-symptoms

- Sudden CONFUSION, trouble speaking or understanding speech.
- Sudden TROUBLE SEEING in one or both eyes.
- Sudden TROUBLE WALKING, dizziness, loss of balance or coordination.
- Sudden SEVERE HEADACHE with no known cause."[89]

A posterior circulation stroke occurs at the back of the brain. Its symptoms are very different from other strokes that normally occur at the front of the brain (anterior circulation strokes) and may also include the following that need immediate attention:

- "Vertigo, like the room, is spinning.
- Imbalance
- One-sided arm or leg weakness.
- Slurred speech or dysarthria (difficulty talking and being understood)
- Double vision or other vision problems
- A headache
- Nausea and/or vomiting"[90]

Now that you know the symptoms, you know to watch for them in yourself and others.

Now let's think:

What would happen to you and your family if you were gone? What would happen if you were hospitalized? What would happen to your chances of these horrible things happening if you could lower your chances of heart disease tenfold by simply getting to a healthy weight? What if you could be a light in the world for a very long time to come? What if you told

---

[89] Learn More Stroke Warning Signs and Symptoms. American Stroke Association. https://www.strokeassociation.org/en/about-stroke/stroke-symptoms/learn-more-stroke-warning-signs-and-symptoms
[90] Ibid.

yourself it would be easy and all of those things that you knew were not good for you would be no longer desirable? Those sweet, salty, fatty, junky foods, that you have been calling treats and rewards, are no longer desirable for you. They mean pain and suffering to you and your family. You can do it. The time is now. A better, healthier you has just begun.

Mental Exercise: Joint Problems and Osteoarthritis.
Read with passion and feeling, or have a friend do so while you close your eyes and visualize:

Too much weight can cause excessive wear and tear on the knees and hips. The extra weight causes extra stress. And while knee and hip replacement surgery may be common these days, they are nothing to plan for. Not only are they surgery, which like any surgery is stressful, but they will also need to be replaced at some point. Right now, they are saying that they last about ten years. It you don't lose weight, however, they may not be even an option because they are not always an advisable option for an obese person.

This is because artificial joints have a higher risk of loosening and causing further damage in those who are obese. But what if you could get rid of that pain by losing weight? Oh, my aching back. What if it could be better if a few pounds were gone? What if it would make your neck, knees, and hips feel better, too?

Osteoarthritis feels like pain and tenderness. Later, it can become more severe and sharp. Your joints feel stiff when you get out of bed, like you don't want to move. It can get better after you get going, but it can be hard. Your joints can click or crack when you move. As the cartilage wears down between the joints, the bones can rub against each other. This can make strange sounds and painful sensations.

You're losing flexibility. The less you move means the less you are able to move. Maybe you can't pick things up off the floor anymore. Or maybe, you can't step into the bathtub. Maybe even turning your head around to back the car out of the driveway is a thing of the past. Maybe your joints lock. They could barely move or not even move at all. At first you may be stiff sometimes, but at the disease gets worse so do the symptoms and the frequency until they are bad all the time. And it may not get better with rest.

But what if the pain could be less, or better yet, if it didn't have to start at all? What if becoming a healthy weight could spare you from a life of discomfort at least, of misery at worst.

What if it is not too late? What if today is a new day? What if weight loss meant freedom of movement and freedom from pain? A life of joyful movement could await. Today is a new day.

The problem with diseases is if you don't think of them, you still get them anyway. Isn't is better to think about them now, while you can hopefully prevent them, rather than waiting until you have them and them trying to cure them. An ounce of prevention is worth a pound of cure (Benjamin Franklin). It is true. Diseases are much easier to prevent than to treat. In this day and age of so-called modern medicine, we seem to think that there is a pill for every ill. Most everybody who takes pills though will tell you that they would rather not take them, and they seldom do the trick entirely. Pain pills seldom take all the pain away, and the pain always seems to come back. So much the better if we could let food be our medicine for both prevention and, if necessary, cure. Better to change our dietary ways than to come under the knife.

Sleep Apnea and Respiratory Problems.

Sleep apnea is one of those things you hear about on the news, but few of us give it much credence. Let's think more about this condition that can be related to much more serious problems. Think with feeling or have a friend read to you as you visualize.

Sleep apnea causes you to stop breathing for brief periods during the night. It interrupts sleep and causes you to be sleepy all day long. Your spouse is sick of it. You may not notice your heavy snoring but she or he certainly does. Your partner can barely stand sleeping in the same room anymore. The snoring is keeping him or her awake. This could explain why you fall asleep while watching television and are tired all day long even when you slept all night. The doctor told you to lose weight, but how can you exercise when you feel like you have no energy?

You know that the excess weight is squeezing the walls of the chest, compressing the lungs, and causing restricted breathing even while awake. Apnea is also associated with high blood pressure, and you know that has all kinds of other problems.

In addition to the snoring and daytime sleepiness, you might also have insomnia and nightmares. It seems like even though you are tired, you can't get to sleep. Your partner reports that he or she is afraid for you, too. Sometimes you actually stop breathing. You may feel that you breathe loudly or have to breathe through the mouth.

In addition, your mouth is dry and your throat. You might also be depressed, fatigued, headachy, irritable, and moody.

When you snore, the sound produced by vibrations in the upper respiratory airways. Part of the airway is blocked as air tries to flow through.

The worrisome part is when breathing stops. This is the part that is labeled apnea. Not everyone who snores has apnea, but if you snore loudly, it is likely.

When you stop breathing the oxygen in your blood drop. Your brain feels this and makes you wake-up, so it can start you breathing again. You may not be aware of this, but the quality of your sleep will be poor, and your normal sleep cycles will be disrupted including your deep REM sleep. You may not realize it, but you may have these episodes even hundreds of times a night! No wonder you feel tired all the time and sleep feels like a chore.

Naps don't make it better either and trying to concentrate can be very difficult. It can even come to the point that driving or operating machinery is out of the question. People with sleep apnea are two to four times more likely to have car accidents.[91]

The lack of oxygen to your head can give you morning headaches to boot making it even harder to cope. Sleep apnea is related to high blood pressure, heart disease, and diabetes, and possibly heart burn and asthma.

So, what is the alternative? A breathing mask and a hose keeping positive air pressure in your lungs to keep things flowing? What about

---

[91] Strohl K, Bonnie R, Findley L, et al. (1994) Sleep apnea, sleepiness, and driving risk. Am J Respir Crit Care Med 150:1463–1473.

sleeping with that? What about the noise the machine generates? What is your partner going to think of that? Intimacy with a breathing mask on? What if losing weight was the answer? For many people that is all it takes. Less fat around the throat, chest, and belly can make breathing easier and may be all it takes to feel like a new, energetic person each and every morning. A new you is on the way. A lighter, refreshed you is the answer.

In addition, high blood pressure can be linked to sleep apnea as well. What if losing weight could help? If you are experiencing apnea, when your brain makes you wake-up due to lack of oxygen it can cause an increase in the pressure in the blood vessels as blood is forced through your veins to get the needed oxygen. Repeated episodes of apnea increase the times when your blood pressure is spiked until that same high blood pressure occurs during the day as well.

That excess weight, including any excess weight around your neck and throat, can cause tissues to fall back into the throat blocking airways which cause the apnea episodes.

We have measured our neck circumferences already and know that if neck circumference is greater than 17 inches for men or 16 inches for women you have a higher risk of sleep apnea because of fatty tissue surrounding your airways which can cause restrictions in breathing during sleep.

Problems with sleep can cause irritability, depression, anxiety, and mood swings. Having a poor night's sleep even one night can be enough to make some people grumpy. When sleeping turns into a night of trying to sleep and constantly waking-up, it can be enough to affect anyone's mood and overall health.

Things can change though. I now know many more things are related to my weight than I ever thought. Knowing these things will give me power. The power to tell myself the right things to do - not just when I am feeling good, but when I feel mentally weak or at my worst. I know that I was not put here to be weak. I was made to be a help to myself and others. I will not make myself a burden to my family by knowingly trying to hurt my future-self. I do not have the excuse of ignorance anymore. I know what is unhealthy and being too heavy certainly cannot be. I am changing. I am improving. I am getting better, healthier and healthier every day!

<u>Cancer.</u>
What an awful, horrible word? Who, in what family, has not been affected? How nice it would be to return to the days of our youth when cancer was but a sign of the zodiac!

Knowing the enemy is the first step in defeating it. This one is tough though, and like some people that are just always trouble, they are better avoided than confronted. Did your mother tell you to always confront the bully, no matter how big or how crazy he was? My mom taught me to know my own strengths, but also know my weaknesses. Why would I want to confront someone who would pummel me even with the law standing right there? The law may get them, but I would still be in for a world of hurt.

I think that it is the same way with cancer. Why would I want to tempt fate by knowingly doing things that are related to its occurrence? It is so easy to claim ignorance and say that fate will have its time and there is nothing you can do about it because your fate is written into your genes. It is so easy to say that everything causes cancer and that there is nothing that you can to. It is so easy to listen to the media hype and proclaim that there is no one who knows what they are talking about and that the scientists cannot agree.

Yes, scientific research is never perfect, but it also is always progressing. Because we have scientific review, because we have ongoing research, we have the best knowledge we can at this moment.

Before my father had esophageal cancer, I was ignorant to the risk factors for this version of the disease. Burning hot coffee, burning hot soup, esophageal reflux, and scotch did him no good. Also, having his chest split open and having his esophagus cut out did him no good either. The re-sectioning left him with holes in his throat. He could either die from infection due to food entering his chest cavity upon re-feeding or die from slow starvation on IV fluids. He was deemed to "old" for additional surgery to open his chest back up, and by the time a port was opened to supply more nutrients than the IV, it was too late. He essentially starved to death after too aggressive surgery. He had stage one cancer. A family friend was diagnosed with stage four esophageal cancer at the same time. He had lung cancer earlier in life and decided this time, as an old man, to do nothing. He lived for eighteen months. My father was dead in two.

I know cancer is a hard thing to think about, but you must know your enemy. You must understand that there is no magic bullet against this one and there may never be, since it has so many variants. Doctors may not be able to save you, but researchers, epidemiologists in particular, may be able to tell you how to steer clear at least until you are very old, and very gray.

Why all this in a weight loss book? Because I love you, and if fear of cancer is going to be what it takes to get you to lose weight, by all means, use this evildoer to your advantage. Being overweight significantly contributes to your risk of many cancers. There is no excuse in ignorance anymore. The life of your future-self is in your hands. This is the end of ignorance and the start to a new healthier, slimmer you.

If you are a woman, if you are overweight you are at increased risk for:

- breast cancer,
- colon cancer,
- gallbladder cancer,
- uterine cancer,
- and possibly endometrial cancer
- and ovarian cancer.

If you are a man, if you are overweight, you are at increased risk for:

- colon cancer
- and prostate cancer.

Both men and women may also be at risk for:

- kidney cancer,
- esophageal cancer,

- gallbladder cancer,
- and pancreatic cancer.

Each of these diseases is a horror in itself, but it is important to know about the signs, symptoms, and consequences of these diseases so that we can at least try to prevent them. I am going to go into some detail about each of these conditions, but please do not confuse these exercises with a medical textbook, that is they will not give you full knowledge of the subject. Instead think of them as mental exercises to get you motivated and say, "I never want anything remotely like that to happen to me (or anyone else for that matter)! Diet makes a difference in prevention. I can get to a healthy weight and help decrease my risk of that horrible disease at least for one thing I can change!"

Yes, you can change. A healthy weight is not too far away. Others have done it and you can do it, too!

<u>Mental Incentive: Thinking About Cancer and Your Risk.</u>
Read the following, then have a friend help you through a visualization if you like:

What if you had cancer? Would you beat it? How long would you battle it? How sick would you be? Would you have surgery? Would you be disfigured? Would you have to have reconstructive surgery? Would the surgery even work? Would you even wake up?

What about chemotherapy? Would you lose your hair? Just how sick might you be? Would your spouse stay and take care of you? Would you have to have a nurse come in to help? What about radiation? Would you even let your kids see you when you are sick, or might they have to live the rest of their lives knowing that they never got to say goodbye?

If you get breast cancer, it can present as swelling on part or all of your breast, nipple discharge, skin soreness, scaly skin, redness, skin thickening, or the nipple turning inward. You can also have swelling in the arm, armpit, or collar bone. And of course, pain and the potential of disfigurement, not to mention death.

Colorectal cancer can cause changes in your bowels and their consistency, excessive gas, blood in your stool, and abdominal and rectal pain. As with most cancers, you can be anemic causing fatigue and susceptibility to infection.

Most people with gallbladder cancer have abdominal pain, nausea, vomiting. Your skin can be yellow (jaundiced), as can the whites of your eyes. This is from the bile building up in the gallbladder. You can feel lumps in your stomach. You can have a swollen stomach, itchy skin, fever, dark urine, and oily bowel movements. Unfortunately, gallbladder cancer can often spread to the liver.

In uterine cancer, women can experience irregular vaginal bleeding including bleeding after menopause or other vaginal discharge. You can have pain or feel like you have a mass or lump in your pelvic area.

Prostate cancer can cause swelling, sensitivity, nausea, and odor. It can also cause a burning sensation when you urinate or, in the early stages, no symptoms at all. Later, you may have the need to urinate urgently. It can also cause terrible pain since it can spread to the spine. The National Cancer Institute lists possible indicators of prostate cancer as "frequent urination especially at night, not being able to urinate, trouble starting to urinate or trouble holding back urination, a weak or interrupted urine flow, pain or a burning feeling during urination, difficulty having an erection, pain during ejaculation, blood in the semen or in the urine, and frequent pain or stiffness in the lower back, hips, or upper thighs." If you are experiencing any of these, by all means, contact your doctor. Now we know some of what can happen, and as with all of these, the result can be extreme pain and death.

Endometrial cancer, as with uterine cancer, may cause unusual vaginal bleeding, pelvic pain, and feeling a mass in your pelvis. Unfortunately, since these symptoms might not be perceived as troublesome, treatment is often delayed, and the likelihood of successful treatment can be diminished.

Kidney cancer can cause blood in the urine causing it to be pink, red, or brown, but not all sufferers present with this. Sufferers may experience low back pain or pain in their side. It may be sudden or nagging. They might feel a lump in the abdomen or a bulge under the skin, but again these may not be noticeable. Anemia is common as is fatigue both from the disease and from the treatment. You can feel short of breath, dizzy, look pale, or have a fever. As with other cancers, you might experience a sudden, unexpected weight loss. While this may be welcome, any weight loss that is sudden and unexpected should be investigated by a physician. Even interest in food can diminish or even go away altogether as cancer spreads.

Esophageal cancer is cancer of the throat. It may present as difficulty or pain when trying to swallow. Any food that is chunky may be particularly difficult. During the disease you may have to eat only pureed foods or liquids. These may also prove to be impossible to swallow as the cancer grows and blocks the pathway to the stomach. You might also experience heart burn, pressure in your chest, choking, coughing, hoarseness, pain in the chest or throat, or vomiting.

One of the first symptoms of pancreatic cancer can be yellowed skin and eyes (jaundice) since they can block the bile duct from the gallbladder. The urine may be brown and bowel movements may be oily, float, or be pale in color or gray. Unfortunately, pancreatic cancer may not be detected until it has spread. Your skin may also itch and your stomach or back ache. You may be nauseous and vomit. We have also heard of drugs for DVT blood clots being advertised lately. These deep vein thrombosis clots can cause pain, swelling, redness, and a warm sensation in veins of the leg. DVT can also be one of the first signs of pancreatic cancer. Pancreatic cancer can cause diabetes if it destroys the insulin producing cells. It can cause a strange appearance to the fat under the skin. The growth of certain tumors can create excessive hormones such as gastrin which can cause stomach ulcers or glucagon which can also cause diabetes, diarrhea, and weight loss. It can also cause a rash that swells and blisters. Some tumors can make insulin causing you to feel tired, confused, sweat, and breathe rapidly. Some tumors make somatostatin causing your stomach to hurt, and you to feel weak, have diarrhea, or be jaundiced. Other hormones can also be produced causing their own equally bad symptoms.

Any cancer can spread, metastasize. As they spread to different organs, they cause their own different symptoms. Spreading to bone can cause extreme pain.

What if there was something you could do now to protect your future-self? What if you could show yourself that you love them and don't want them to suffer? What if eating healthier now was the key? What if you were one of those fortunate people that did not have to suffer if you reduced your risk of cancer by achieving a healthy weight? What if the end of life did not mean undue, prolonged suffering? What if not eating something meant that you could live longer? Other people have done it! You can do it too!

Metabolic Syndrome.

Metabolic Syndrome is found in one third of all overweight or obese people in the U.S. It is a risk factor for cardiovascular disease and includes abdominal (visceral) obesity, elevated blood cholesterol, elevated blood pressure, insulin resistance with or without glucose intolerance (diabetes), elevated markers of inflammation, and elevated specific clotting factors in the blood.

Losing weight decreases your risk of metabolic syndrome and its associated cardiovascular risk. Going vegan can lower your weight, bring your cholesterol into a healthy range, control your blood pressure, improve your insulin response and even reverse diabetes, and lower markers of inflammation and abnormally high clotting factors. Going vegan could give you a lot less things to worry about.

You can take a few minutes now and visualize this on your own. Think about how metabolic syndrome might affect you and what you can do to help avoid it.

Gallbladder Disease and Gallstones.

Gallbladder disease and gallstones are other problems that you are less likely to face if you maintain a healthy weight. Many times, people with gallstone have no symptoms, but when they do, expect stomach pain, back pain, and even shoulder pain that may be severe. You may think that you are having a heart attack. If gallstones block a bile duct, the pain can be severe with fever and chills. Your skin or whites of your eyes can be yellow. With gallbladder disease you may have nausea and vomiting, heart burn, gas, fever, and chills. If you have more than four bowel movements per day for at least three months, this should be checked by a physician as a potential symptom. Light colored stool and dark urine should be checked as well.

How nice to have a lower risk by being a good weight! What a great reason to be vegan! Again take time to visualize and internalize this information.

<u>Gout.</u>
The first time I heard of gout was in studying the gluttonous eating habits of the wealthy, obese English royalty. Unbeknownst to me, my middle school mind thought it was a disease of the past, long gone with the American Revolution. However, gout is something that is still here, but thankfully something that you as new healthy weight vegan will never be likely to get.

Gout is a joint disorder caused by a buildup of uric acid crystals. The uric acid is from the breakdown of purines (proteins) found in foods, especially meat. Not only do the uric acid crystals cause painful arthritis-like symptoms, but they can also cause kidney stones, kidney blockage, and kidney failure. The joints may feel warm, swollen, and painful. The big toe joint of the foot is commonly affected as are the ankles, knees, fingers, wrists, and elbows. Even touching these joints may cause severe pain and the attacks may last anywhere from hours to weeks.

What a great thing to help yourself avoid by being a healthy weight veggie!

<u>Breathing Problems and Asthma.</u>
Did you know, the overweight and obese are more likely to suffer breathing problems and asthma? Obesity hypoventilation syndrome (a.k.a. Pickwickian Syndrome) is caused by excess fat on your neck, chest, or midsection making it difficult to breathe. The weight of the fat can compress your lungs, throat, diaphragm, and chest, thus restricting the amount of air that you can take in, your lung volume. Fat is an active tissue hormonally, and these hormones can adversely affect your breathing as well. Sleep apnea is often related. Obesity hypoventilation syndrome can make it difficult to breathe and

get enough oxygen. You also have to spend excess energy just on breathing and get tired easily. You may also have headaches, snore, and feel out of breath. Your doctor can check for this condition by measuring you blood oxygen and carbon dioxide levels. If you notice any of these symptoms, they should be brought to your doctor's attention. These can be related to high blood pressure, heart failure, and erythrocytosis (increase red blood cell mass) which can lead to blood clots, heart attack, stroke, and increased risk for leukemia and other blood cancers.[92] [93]

As far as asthma, the research is not clear. While it appears that there are more people that are obese that have asthma and that losing weight can improve asthma symptoms, current research does not show causation.[94] The systemic inflammation that is a result of obesity has been thought to play a significant role. Overweight people are 1.38 times more likely to have asthma than normal weight people and obese people 1.92 times more likely to have asthma than normal weight people.[95] Obese asthmatics may also feel that they have less control of their condition. This is complicated by the fact that inhaled steroids are less effective in obese asthmatics than normal weight asthmatics.[96]

We have done a lot of visualizations together thus far in this book. Take the opportunity here to do one concerning your breathing now on your own. Start with visualizing the

---

[92] National Heart, Lung, and Blood Institute. Obesity Hypoventilation Syndrome. https://www.nhlbi.nih.gov/health-topics/obesity-hypoventilation-syndrome
[93] Watson, Stephanie. Erythrocytosis. Healthline. Jan 16, 2018. https://www.healthline.com/health/erythrocytosis
[94] Ford, Earl S. The epidemiology of obesity and asthma. The Journal of allergy and Clinical Immunology. May 2005. https://doi.org/10.1016/j.jaci.2004.11.050
[95] Beuther, David A., Sutherland, E.Rand. Overweight, Obesity, and Incident Asthma, A meta-analysis of prospective epidemiologic studies. Am J Respir Crit Care Med. 2007 Apr 1; 175(7): 661–666.
[96] Asthma and Obesity. Asthma Initiative of Michigan. For Healthy Lungs. https://getasthmahelp.org/asthma-obesity.aspx

negative and be sure to end with visualizing the positive. We always want to end on a positive note to keep us motivated and happy. There is no point being a sad vegan. Be happy and healthy. Don't feel guilty and sad. Better days are to come!

<u>Pregnancy Problems.</u>

Female? Obese? Haven't had a baby yet or want to have another one? Obese women are more likely to have high blood sugar and gestational diabetes when pregnant. They also have a greater risk of high blood pressure. This can turn into pre-eclampsia (high blood pressure and protein in the urine that can be fatal for both the mother and infant) and eclampsia (a rare advanced form including seizures) causing a profound risk of serious complications for both the mother and infant. Because of these problems and difficulty in delivery in general there is an increased risk for cesarean delivery. C-sections are not ideal. They pose their own risks. They are surgery and do take a long time to recuperate from.

Becoming healthier before pregnancy is ideal. It makes pregnancy easier for both the mother and the infant. Very many complications of pregnancy can be simplified, if not eliminated, by a healthy diet. Achieving a healthy weight before pregnancy is much better than simply trying not to gain too much weight while you are pregnant. Making yourself healthier with natural, lifegiving fruits, vegetables, whole grains, beans, and legumes allows the environment to be the best before establishing a new life. Pregnancy has enough going on without having to worry about things that you wouldn't have to if you achieved a healthy weight beforehand.

If you want to have a baby, I am sure that you have thought about these things extensively. Take the time now to visualize a positive, healthy, happy future.

<u>Psychosocial Effects</u>

I'm sure that I don't have to tell you that being overweight has serious psychological and social consequences. Being obese can make matters much worse. Even having too much weight in a particular spot can cause problems. Ever been asked when you were due? Carrying your weight on your stomach can be a pain in the butt!

Socially, doing thing with people who are not your same weight can be difficult. In school, kids can be cruel with torment. Just getting around, sitting in seats whether in a theater, bus, plane, or doctor's office can be a challenge sometimes. Just finding a spot to sit down when shopping or needing to sit down can be physically tiresome and psychologically discouraging.

One can't help but feel psychological effects. Trying to lose weight time and time again can sometimes make one just want to forget it. Why try to deprive yourself when it doesn't seem to help anyway? Bias and discrimination may be intended as torment and nastiness. Needling may be well intended but can lead to depression and nihilistic tendencies, as well. Why should anything matter and why should you try to improve?

Well, I think you know by now, you should not be depressed, and life is worth living. It is my hope, that by sharing the stories of people just like all of us, you can find hope, a goal, and a plan for becoming a healthier you. Weight loss is an on-going psychological battle. Do not give in. This is a new day. Take e time now to visualize a happier you and carry that spirit into the future.

CHAPTER 4

RECLAIMING YOUR HEALTH PHYSICALLY &
MENTALLY

SUMMARY

- Being too heavy can cause serious health problems
  both now and in the future.
- By knowing the consequences of being overweight, we
  can help to mentally condition ourselves work to
  eliminate current poor health conditions and/or to
  avoid problems in the future.

5 REFINING YOUR DIET

I lost 100 pounds by adopting a vegetarian, and then vegan diet, and exercise program. I'm proud of my accomplishment!

<u>You Are Not What You Do Just One Day.</u>
You are what you do most days. They used to say, if you eat something, it would be part of you for seven years. What are you made out of? Are you mostly white sugar, white flour, chicken fat, and meat? Or are you whole grains, fruit, and vegetables? If you eat foods that are living, doesn't it make sense that you would feel more living yourself? If you are used to eating sugar and flour with all of the nutrients removed, is it any wonder that you want to go to sleep after a meal.

What about that meat? It sits in your stomach. You are not a big cat with stomach acid strong enough to disintegrate it. It sits in your stomach causing heart burn. The reflux is harming your throat. You are not a big cat with a short digestive system that gets rid of the waste quickly. You have a much longer digestive system, perhaps that's why you feel bloated, gaseous, and constipated all the time. Perhaps that is also why colon and rectal cancer are more prevalent among meat eaters. The waste just sits in the system too long. Waste can build up at the end of the colon and harden causing impaction. When this happens you really feel sick with possible abdominal pain, nausea, vomiting, bloating, headache, and liquid leaking. You could even experience your heart racing, heavy breathing, confusion, and incontinence (leaking urine). Impaction means that you must get the waste removed, often manually or with an enema. In any event it is very unpleasant, painful, may cause tears, you won't forget it, and may just do anything to avoid it again. The key to avoidance is plenty of fiber and drinking a lot of water to plump that fiber out and send it through your system. As a vegetarian, and especially as a vegan, almost everything you eat contains fiber. The end of meat means the end of sticky grease in your insides. It also means less likelihood of heart disease,[97] diabetes,[98] colorectal cancer.[99]

Vegetarians have a better antioxidant status than apparently healthy meat-eaters.[100] Obese subject switching to a vegan diet lose weight, lower triglycerides, lower total cholesterol, lower LDL cholesterol, lower A1C, improve fasting glucose, and improve glucose after eating vegan food for just one month.[101] Low-grade inflammation of the intestine caused by intestinal microbes can also cause metabolic dysfunction. Just one month of a vegan diet can increase friendly gut microbes and

---

[97] Huang T, Yang B, Zheng J, Li G, Wahlqvist M.L., Li D. Cardiovascular Disease Mortality and Cancer Incidence in Vegetarians: A Meta-Analysis and Systematic Review. Ann Nutr Metab 2012;60:233–240.

[98] Yoko Yokoyama,Neal D. Barnard, Susan M. Levin, Mitsuhiro Watanabe. Vegetarian diets and glycemic control in diabetes: a systematic review and meta-analysis. Cardiovasc Diagn Ther. 2014 Oct; 4(5): 373–382.

[99] Huand, T. 2012.

[100] Y.T.Szeto PhD, Timothy C.Y.Kwok MD, Iris F.F.Benzie DPhil. Effects of a long-term vegetarian diet on biomarkers of antioxidant status and cardiovascular disease risk. Nutrition. Volume 20, Issue 10, October 2004, Pages 863-866.

[101] Min-Soo Kim, Seong-Soo Hwang, Eun-Jin Park, Jin-Woo Bae. Strict vegetarian diet improves the risk factors associated with metabolic diseases by modulating gut microbiota and reducing intestinal inflammation. Environmental Microbiology Reports. Volume 5, Issue 5. 26 June 2013.

decrease pathogenic ones while reducing intestinal inflammation.[102] My mom said, "When I became vegetarian, I was never constipated again."

<u>Dietary Exercise: My Favorite Foods.</u>
You guessed it. I'm going to ask you to write down your favorite foods here. Let's make a list. You can rank them if you want. If you don't have ten favorite foods, leave some spaces blank. If you have more than ten favorite foods, by all means write them down.

1.

2.

3.

4.

5.

6.

7.

8.

9.

10.

---

[102] Ibid.

Now let's think about them. Which of those foods are healthy? Let's consider our definition of healthy. Are they of plant origin? Are they full of nutrients? Are they minimally processed, if at all?

Is there any way that you could make your favorite foods healthier? Are there any foods you shouldn't eat at all? Put a nice "x" through those foods that maybe you shouldn't eat in the future. Maybe these are foods you may just want to eat once a year at a holiday gathering or birthday. Maybe you don't want to consider them worthy to be made part of your body anymore. Food is not just for energy. It is easy for us to consider a child growing and the foods you feed them becoming part of their bones and muscles. Adults still have turnover of cells. Muscles change. Bones change. You are literally not the same person you were ten years ago. Maybe you don't want to be partially made out of chicken fat any more. Why do I say chicken fat specifically? Well, the population has cut down on a lot of red meat, but most of them have replaced it with chicken. The consumption of chicken (along with pork, "the other white-meat", red meat, other poultry, and processed meat) has been related to increased weight gain (BMI) in both men and women.[103]

Now let's think how we could make some of those favorite

---

[103] Gilsing AM1, Weijenberg MP, Hughes LA, Ambergen T, Dagnelie PC, Goldbohm RA, Brandt PA, Schouten LJ. Longitudinal changes in BMI in older adults are associated with meat consumption differentially, by type of meat consumed. J Nutr. 2012 Feb;142(2):340-9.
Vergnaud AC1, Norat T, Romaguera D, Mouw T, May AM, Travier N, Luan J, Wareham N, Slimani N, Rinaldi S, Couto E, Clavel-Chapelon F, Boutron-Ruault MC, Cottet V, Palli D, Agnoli C, Panico S, Tumino R, Vineis P, Agudo A, Rodriguez L, Sanchez MJ, Amiano P, Barricarte A, Huerta JM, Key TJ, Spencer EA, Bueno-de-Mesquita B, Büchner FL, Orfanos P, Naska A, Trichopoulou A, Rohrmann S, Hermann S, Boeing H, Buijsse B, Johansson I, Hellstrom V, Manjer J, Wirfält E, Jakobsen MU, Overvad K, Tjonneland A, Halkjaer J, Lund E, Braaten T, Engeset D, Odysseos A, Riboli E, Peeters PH. Meat consumption and prospective weight change in participants of the EPIC-PANACEA study. Am J Clin Nutr. 2010 Aug;92(2):398-407.

foods healthier. Could you change the cooking method? Could you make them yourself and use whole wheat flour and less sugar? Could you use a baked or low salt version? Could you eat less of it? Or is it better cut out of our diets altogether? Is the fun of it now not worth the potential pain of it latter?

Now let's make a list of foods that may not be on your list above, but if someone puts them in front of you, if they are available, you will not stop eating them literally until they are gone, or they are physically removed from you. My mom used to do that. There were just some foods I just wouldn't stop eating and she would literally just come and take them away. Mind you, there were other foods I just wouldn't eat, and she would force me to sit at the table until I took "three bites." Anyway, I don't live with my mother anymore, but it still would be good to have someone take certain foods away from me. My alter-ego mother-self inside me seems to appear and take the food away from that gluttonous, ravenous self that wants to keep eating. It is not even that I feel full. There are just some foods that if they are available I will just eat until they are no longer. For me, that is definitely movie-theater popcorn (I will eat all of it and get a headache and bloating afterwards from drinking too much because of the salt) and certain packaged cookies. I try very hard not to eat either of these, popcorn because it makes me feel sick and packaged cookies because I don't want all the junky calories.

What is on your list of foods that if they were put in front of you, you could eat nonstop until they were gone?

1.

2.

3.

4.

5.

Let's think about these foods. Ask yourself if you think they are healthy? Do you think it is good for you to eat them with abandon? Could they actually be good for you? If you can't stop eating a bowl of cherries or a whole cantaloupe, maybe in fact, they are good for you. If they are loaded with salt or fat or sugar, they are not. If you can't stop eating that pack of cookies, maybe you shouldn't have them at all. Maybe that stomachache, headache, or comatose-feeling afterwards is enough to deter you. Maybe you need to think about something else to deter you, like your weight or your health. And sometimes, you just don't care. The trick is to get yourself to care most of the time. You are not what you do some of the time. You are what you do most of the time.

The sign to hell might read: "Abandon all hope yea who enter here." I might add: "Those who eat with abandon, may abandon all hope for the future."

<u>What Were We Taught About Food?</u>
Let's take a minute to think about what we were taught about food. Think about what you were taught about not the content of food, but how food was handled in your home growing-up.

A lot of associations are made in our childhood that we may not realize their origin unless we actively seek to explore them. Let me give you an example unrelated to food. A close relative of mine was raised in a very poor household during the depression. Everything was hard to come by. They had very little, and thus the things they did have became very important and meaningful. Things were worn until they were worn out. As an adult, this same person has all the money that could ever be wanted. Still, they wear things until they are falling apart and hold onto vast amounts of stuff. Things are very difficult to let go of. This may be a good quality. After all, frugality is a good Protestant trait. Waste not, want not, right? But what if this trait brings about hoarding. My mom and I joke about this: "What is the difference between a hoarder and a collector? A collector can afford it." Also, a hoarder might not be able to walk through their house. Indeed, it may be a fire-hazard. It is a matter of degree and perspective. One man's trash is another man's treasure.

Now, let's think about foods. Read the following slowly to yourself, or have a friend read it to you, as you think about your early life with food:

How were you taught about food? What was the attitude about food in your family growing-up? Was it an attitude of abundance or one of scarcity? Did you eat together or separately? Did you eat with the television on or in front of the computer perhaps with a headset on? Did one of your parents make dinner or did you have to find yourself something to eat?

What were your first foods? If your parents are still alive and you don't know, find out. It may be enlightening. How were you fed? Were you forced to eat? Did you make a fuss? Were you a picky eater? Were you forced to stay at the table? Did you have to clear your plate? Were you allowed to throw food out?

Did your family cook? Did you get a lot of take out? Did your family ever bake? Did your family ever have a garden? Did your family feel that food was recreation? Was the main cooking method the microwave? Did you ever help in the kitchen? Did you want to help in the kitchen, but were kicked out?

What did you see your parents and relatives eating? Did they stuff themselves? Did they stop you from eating? Did they fall asleep after eating?

What was the general attitude about food? Did you pray before meals? Did family members view food with reverence? Did anyone have any interesting dietary practices? Was anyone vegetarian? Did they ridicule vegetarians?

How have these early exposures affected your attitude toward eating? How have these early exposures affected your weight?

Let me give you some examples of what may have happened. Really strange things can happen with parents, children, and food. We once had two very overweight boys come in and have the mother say that they did not eat much of anything at all. After much questioning she admitted that she would put everything that they should have eaten during the day into the blender and woke them up in the middle of the night to feed it to them. Other people might have very little in the house, so not eating, no matter how much you as the child did not like the food, was not an option. Some houses may not have a functional parent and children are left to fend for themselves or help younger children. This can amount to children raising themselves or raising other children, their siblings. This may happen for a variety of reasons such as alcohol or drugs, spousal abuse, or even depression. If someone is sick, either physically or mentally, it may be very difficult to take care of yourself much less take care of a child. Then there is the extreme case of child abuse as well.

Hopefully, for most of us, our childhood experiences with food are more mundane. Perhaps, there was little fresh food in the household, or the family never sat down to meals together because everyone was running around trying to get somewhere else. In any event, our childhood experiences can shape the way we look at food for both the good and bad. Give it some thought and write down:

Some good ways that my childhood has influenced what I eat:

____

____

____

And some bad ways that my childhood has influenced what I eat:

____

____

____

What can I do now to change how I feel about those childhood experiences and improve my current diet?

____

____

____

What Were You Taught About Meat?

Unless you were raised a vegetarian, you probably were raised with a lot of feelings about animal products including feelings about people who avoid them. Let's see. You probably heard that vegetarians were health nuts or hippies. You at least heard that they were weird, or maybe wimps that deserved to be picked on. Maybe you heard that they were hippies or druggies. Maybe you said meat was part of your culture or you could never do that.

Meat is part of American culture, but even in the last twenty years it has become less so. Everyone is becoming more aware of the detrimental health effects of too much meat, or at least too little plant products. Things are changing. Germany, who used to be the home of exclusively sausage and potatoes, now has several vegetarian options available in places even like the famous Haufbrau House Beer Hall in Munch. They don't curl up their noses at you anymore when you say you are vegetarian. And now people actually know what vegan means.

So, let's examine what you think about meat. Can you live without it? Is it something you grew up with? Is it something that you could change your feelings about?

The Power of Positive Thinking.

We have been doing a lot of work with negative associations. Let's think of some positive associations now.

Think about the following:

What would you gain with extra years in your life? Would you see your children grow-up and get married? Will you have time to play with your grandkids? Being healthy would add years to your life, but perhaps more importantly, being healthy could add life to your years. Losing weight could mean being able to get down on the floor and play with those grandkids not just being able to see them. It could make the difference between working and being productive or being on disability. Imagine sleeping better at night and waking up refreshed. Imagine being comfortable in your skin. Imagine peace of mind. Think of all the fun things you could do with more energy and health. Imaging the outfits and looking good. Hear the compliments. Feel the joy of being able to move. Picture the beauty of the outdoors and you as one of God's creatures living joyfully, feeling the sun on your happy, smiling face and the breeze on your skin. Imagine feeling able to suck in your stomach and have not much of anything there. Imagine less doctor's visits and fewer medical bills. Imagine health for the rest of your life. You can do this. Meat is worth giving up.

So Why Follow a Risky Diet When You Can Lose Weight on a Perfectly Safe One?

That is a great question to ask yourself: "Why would I want to ingest foods which raise my risks of serious disease?" I know I wouldn't. I love myself and my family too much to put my health at risk. So, the question is: Can I get all the nutrients I need, be healthy, and still lose weight?

Overwhelmingly, yes! In fact, you have the potential to be much healthier than you are right now! There are a multitude of foods to eat and becoming a vegan opens doors to new tastes, ethnicities, and combinations that you may have otherwise avoided because you were stuck in your meat and potatoes rut.

Take the Healthy Diet and Life-Style Quiz

With so any weight loss programs out there, how can you possibly know where to start? It can be so overwhelming. You may just want to give up before you even begin. I've given you a lot to think about, but let's think about ourselves a little more by means of this fun quiz.

Don't stress. Stress can make you eat more. So, let's start at the very beginning! Let's find out all about you. Let's see how you are doing, what your needs are, what your goals are or should be, and how it best suits you, as an individual, to meet and maintain your achievements.

Don't worry! It's fun and you just might learn a lot about yourself on the way.

Circle your answers and be honest with yourself. Let's go!

1) How would you characterize your diet?
   a. I consciously eat a variety of foods on a daily basis.
   b. I eat what is available to me at the time and don't really think about what I am eating.
   c. I try to watch what I eat, but usually don't have much time to devote to what I eat.

2) Which do you do?
   a. I always read labels and choose foods accordingly.
   b. I never read food labels and don't change my diet based on a food label.
   c. I don't really know how to use a food label but may change my diet if I understood more about the content of foods.

3) I eat:
   a. Five or more fruits and vegetables a day.
   b. Maybe three or four fruits and vegetables a day.
   c. Maybe one or two fruits and vegetables a day.
   d. Maybe one fruit or vegetable every other day.
   e. Fruit or vegetables hardly ever.

4) I eat:
   a. Dark green vegetables almost every day.
   b. Dark green vegetables once a week.
   c. As few dark green vegetables as humanly possible.

5) I eat orange and yellow fruits and vegetables:
   a. Almost every day.
   b. At least once or twice a week.

c. Never.

6) How often do you eat whole grains?
   a. Three or more times a day.
   b. Once a day.
   c. A few times a week.

7) I avoid trans fatty acids.
   a. True.
   b. False.
   c. I don't know what they are.

8) I have tracked the amount of cholesterol in my diet.
   a. True.
   b. False.

9) I eat deep fried foods.
   a. True.
   b. False.

10) I eat whole milk dairy products like ice cream and whole milk.
    a. True.
    b. False.

11) When I bake, I use white flour.
    a. True.
    b. False.
    c. I only use a mix.

12) How much cholesterol do you get in your diet?
    a. Zero.
    b. Less than 300 mg per day.
    c. Probably more than 300 mg per day.
    d. I have no idea.

What an easy quiz! Let's talk about your answers.

First off, there are no right and wrong answers to this quiz. No one is grading you. This is just a self-exploratory exercise for you to think more about how healthy you are eating right now.

You probably don't need me to tell you the right answers, do you?

If you watch the news, or even just talk to people, you have a pretty good idea that you should:

1. Eat a variety of foods.
2. Eat a bunch of fruit and vegetable daily.
3. Eat dark green, orange, and yellow fruits and vegetables.
4. Eat whole grains.
5. Avoid cholesterol, trans fats, and deep frying.
6. And, skip the high fat dairy and white flour.

Most of us have heard to follow these guidelines. The problem is that many of us don't follow them.

Let's think about each of these items some more.

How would you characterize your diet? Like most of us this question probably depends on what day it is. For now, you should start to try thinking about consciously eating a variety of foods on a daily basis. Most of what you eat should be from plants and have as little processing as possible. If you eat only what is available, this could turn out well or not. Try at this point to start thinking about what you are eating. Think about what you are about to put in your mouth and make it a conscious decision what you eat. If you just shove things in your mouth as you go about other business, your diet is never going to have the importance in your life as the giver of life, health, and longevity that it truly is. (Spoken like a real nutritionist, right?)

A lot of people pray before meals. This is a great habit to get into whether you are religious or not. If you lay out everything you are going to eat before you eat it, only what you have laid out for your meal should be consumed. The Hare

Krishnas (and other religions, too) do not take even a bite to taste while they are cooking. They cannot eat anything before everything is blessed. Praying, breathing deeply, or any other mindful activity to settle yourself before a meal brings you into the moment, relaxes you, and helps the meal be more enjoyable and calmer. There should be no hurry to mealtime. Sometimes when you want to eat when you are rushed, you just might be better off not eating at all if you eat without thinking and feel dissatisfied afterwards only to overeat again later.

Many Jews take it a step further and pray at the end of the meal as well. What a nice way to say thank you to the universe and tell yourself it is time to stop.

If you're trying to watch what you eat, but don't have much time to think about it, going vegetarian is a great way to go, vegan even better. By picking items on a menu or in a store with these labels, you will automatically be picking healthier options than the typical fatty, meaty fare. Most places these days have a veggie burger, which has got to be healthier than other burgers on the menu. Even ordering a cheese pizza is going to be better than a ground beef or pepperoni, and one with veggies would be even better.

Which do you do: I always read labels and choose foods accordingly? I never read food labels and don't change my diet based on a food label? I don't really know how to use a food label but may change my diet if I understood more about the content of foods? Guess what? I think that there is always more to learn when it comes to food labeling. If you feel overwhelmed, you're not alone. Reading labels can hurt your eyes and leave you so frustrated especially if you're trying to shop in a hurry or are distracted (like when the kids come along and ask for everything). The good news is though, you only really have to read food labels once (although sometimes ingredients do change especially when the packaging changes.) Don't force yourself to read a whole label before you put something new back on the shelf. Make yourself a mental list of what you won't eat. Scan the label and if the food contains something you won't eat, it is not a food for you.

Guess where vegetarians get their name! They are supposed to eat a lot of vegetables! Silly? Go ahead and eat fruits and grains. They are from plants, too. But one of the things that make vegetarian really healthy is eating a lot of vegetables. You could make yourself an unhealthy vegetarian, too. I call that a health-food, junk-food vegetarian. Relying on prepackaged vegetarian junk may not be great, but if you were a real junk-food, fatty food, deep-fried meat junky before, it may be just what you need. Anyway, find some vegetables and eat them. If you don't eat any dark green vegetables or any of those from the cabbage family, they are some of the best ones to include to help your future-self avoid the pain of cancers later on.[104] Try some cabbage, broccoli, cauliflower, Brussels sprouts, kale, collard greens, beet greens, Swiss chard, or radishes. A lot of these are incorporated into green juices these days, too. Just don't drink too much of these store prepared brands. Most of them are mainly fruit juice which can add a lot of calories to your diet if you gulp them down unconsciously. Try to limit these to a cup or so a day. Drinking too many calories can be very easy to do. Find some vegetables that you like and eat them. The fiber that was removed from juicing will do you good. Whole foods will help fill you up and keep your colon moving along.

If you really hate vegetables, don't worry. Fruits provide many of the same benefits. Peaches, nectarines, plums, and cherries have all been linked to lowered cancer risk. Again, try to eat them in their whole state. You could easily drink ten oranges in a glass of orange juice that you could never finish if you ate them whole.

Another group of fruits and vegetables that is often overlooked are those that are deep orange and yellow, or dark green. These include carrots, sweet potato, kale, spinach, dark leafy greens, winter squash, cantaloupe, and apricots. These are

---

[104] JW Fahey, KK Stephenson. Cancer chemoprotective effects of cruciferous vegetables. HortScience, Vol 34(7): 1999.

the ones that are high in beta-carotene that have been shown to decrease cancer risk.[105] Beta-carotene turns into Vitamin A in your system and vitamin supplements have not always been shown in every study to have the same effect.

Depending on who you have been reading lately, don't let them give you any hogwash about whole grains. Yes, we should be eating whole grains multiple times a day. Our ancestors would not have had much to eat if it weren't for them, and by that, I mean your not so distant grandparents, not your Neanderthal relatives. Whole grains are a staple of the diet. They are full of vitamins, minerals, and energy. Whole grains mean grain without the bran and germ of the grain removed. These are the parts especially high in nutrients including fats. Without the bran and germ, most bugs won't even eat them. Whole grains should include any grains that you like including wheat, rice, spelt, kamut, sorghum, oats, barley, buckwheat, corn, amaranth, etc. Don't be fooled by the whole anti-gluten fad, too. Unless you have been tested and are truly allergic or sensitive to gluten, you're probably not. Skipping gluten isn't something you can just do a few times a day, or even a few days a week. People who are truly sensitive to gluten must avoid it. It takes time for the gut lining to heal and gluten must be avoided, down to even the few grains of gluten that your gluten-free toast may pick-up on the toaster from the last piece of wheat bread toasted. Very many gluten-free foods are also "halo-foods." That is, they are junk foods with junky other ingredients basking in the glow of the latest health food label. If you think you are sensitive to gluten, by all means get tested. In fact, get tested for everything. There are at-home, finger-stick, blood food sensitivity tests you can take and send in to be analyzed. I speak from experience when I say, finding unknown food allergies, and eliminating them, can make a huge difference in your health.

---

[105] R. Peto, R. Doll, J. D. Buckley & M. B. Sporn. Can dietary beta-carotene materially reduce human cancer rates? Nature. Volume 290, pages201–208 (1981).

One thing I will say about grains is since you're interested in weight loss, you should be conscious of serving sizes. Gorging on bowl after bowl of pasta or eating whole loaves of bread won't help no matter how "whole" your grains are. A good trick is to use a measuring cup as your serving utensil. That way, you know just how much you are taking, and other members of the family can take just how much they want, too. A friend of mine taught me this trick. She told me every time I cooked by eye, especially baked, I should use measuring cups and spoons rather than just dumping ingredients in. That way I could always tell other people what I did and replicate my recipes. Thanks, Diane.

On to the next question. The majority of trans-fats are produced when hydrogen is pumped through a liquid oil to make it more solid margarine. Interestingly, the negative health effects of trans-fatty acids on heart disease were discovered in Israeli populations of Jews using vegetable margarines for keeping Kosher. This is one case in which vegetarian does not necessarily mean healthier. If you are trying to lose weight, limiting the amount of solid fat in any form that you spread on bread, cook with, or eat in processed foods is a good idea. The federal government is limiting the use of hydrogenated fats/trans-fatty acids in processed foods and has required companies to reformulate their products or petition to permit their use in specific cases.[106] Naturally occurring trans fats, however, are still present in small amounts in meats and dairy.[107] I opt for extra virgin olive oil. The most long-lived populations in the world, the Ikarians of Greece and the Sardinians of Italy, use this for both eating and cooking. Canola oil and soy oil are also used by the Okinawans, also famed for their longevity. Canola, by the way, comes from rapeseed which is a crucifer.

If you are one of those vegans that opts for "fake" cheeses, please start reading the label. Many of these products are

---

[106] Tans Fat. FDA website.
https://www.accessdata.fda.gov/scripts/interactivenutritionfactslabel/trans-fat.html
[107] Ibid.

primarily processed oils. Anytime a food is highly processed it takes the body less energy to process. For example, processed cereals are processed grain that is cooked and then pushed through an extruder as mush to form a shape as they are exposed to very high temperatures to cook again and solidify. Is it any wonder that most cereals turn to mush in milk? They are pre-cooked, hardened mush anyway. Is it also any wonder that they take practically no energy for your body to digest and assimilate? The more you cook and process any food, the less there is for your body to do. If you are a cereal junkie, try this: Give it up. Pick something that you have to chew. Shredded wheat is better than puffed shapes even if they say they are whole grain and say they supply a day's supply of whatever. The same goes for those cheeses. Read the ingredients. Maybe having a handful of nuts might be a better idea?

People used to think that everything about heart disease was about cholesterol. Today, scientific thinking has changed, but don't let them tell you that populations that eat a lot of cholesterol are healthier. They are not. Blood cholesterol can be related to a number of factors and your body does make its own. Cholesterol, however, only comes in animal products. If you are vegan, you are not eating any. And if you are vegan, you probably are eating more folic acid than the average meat eater.[108] Folic acid intake is significantly inversely related to cholesterol levels and heart disease rates. This has been known for a long time.[109] Vegetarians are not a population know to get heart disease. So, eat your veggies and skip the cholesterol!

I'm sure you know that many people feel deep fat frying can make anything taste better. True, right down to my pappy's

---

[108] Leitzmann C. Vegetarian Diets: What Are the Advantages? Diet Diversification and Health Promotion. Forum Nutr. Basel, Karger, 2005, vol 57, pp 147-156. https://doi.org/10.1159/000083787
[109] Carol J. Boushey, PhD, MPH, RD; Shirley A. A. Beresford, PhD; Gilbert S. Omenn, MD, PhD; et al. A Quantitative Assessment of Plasma Homocysteine as a Risk Factor for Vascular Disease, Probable Benefits of Increasing Folic Acid Intakes. JAMA. 1995;274(13):1049-1057. doi:10.1001/jama.1995.03530130055028

old rubber boot. That doesn't mean it is good for you though. Deep fat frying adds a lot of calories to anything. Frying is a drying reaction. That is, water goes out, a browning reaction occurs, and some fat is absorbed. I'm sure your know that high temperature frying breaks down the fat and creates harmful polymeric and oxidized material by-products as the fat deteriorates.[110] What you may not be aware of though is how most restaurants handle frying. Number one, they fry in the least expensive oil possible. They are not going to fry in extra virgin olive oil that they use one or two times and then throw out. Extra virgin olive oil only presses the olives and uses no chemicals or heat for extraction. If they use olive oil, they are going to use pomace olive oil which extracts the most oil possible out of those guys though the use of a hexane solvent and refining with acids, bases, and heat. They more likely use a "vegetable" oil and by that you can read that it is so cheap and chemically extracted that they don't even want to call it something recognizable like corn or soy bean oil. They just use a mix of whatever of vegetable origin that is least expensive at the time. This can certainly include cottonseed oil. Now when was the last you fried up some good cotton seeds for dinner. Not exactly food, right? Despite all these cost savings, oil is one of the most expensive food stuffs they buy in food service. Now since restaurants have bought all this expensive oil and have to fill huge fryers with it, they are not going to dump it the way you would if you had saved some fat to use the next day and changed your mind about using it again after you caught a whiff of its putrid smell. Commercial fryers have built in filters and in order to use them you first have to dump in their special mix of chemicals. They cause the dirt floating in the vat of oil to settle to the bottom so it can then be filtered out. These chemicals are not foods, but they will tell you that they will be filtered out. To me, that is why my husband always

---

[110] E. G. PerkinsL. A. van Akkeren. Heated fats. IV. Chemical changes in fats subjected to deep fat frying processes: Cottonseed oil. Journal of the American Oil Chemists Society. September 1965, Volume 42, Issue 9, pp 782–786.

seems to get digestive problems when we eat out. Most restaurant quality oil is terrible. If you are going to do some frying, please do it at home with minimal oil to limit calories. Do it quickly to limit the amount of oil the food soaks up, but with low enough a temperature to prevent burning. Finally, by all means, throw out oils after a use or two. And as we are trying to lose weight, limit them to a once in a great while as a treat. Again, your taste buds will adjust so that fatty fried foods will have a greasy mouth-feel the less you eat them. The less of them you eat, when you do eat them you'll just feel like you have to go brush your teeth to get that greasy coating out of your mouth.

Are you a baby cow? If you answered yes, go ahead and keep eating whole milk dairy products. If not, maybe drinking milk and eating cheese isn't helping you in your weight loss plans. Milk was made to grow an average 83 pound calf into a 1,000 to 1,800 pound cow or 1,900 to 2,2000 pound bull. Humans are the only animal in which all of us don't wean. Other animal mothers don't let their offspring continue. While milk and cheese may be part of culture or have helped humans live in conditions and climates in which they may have otherwise not have been able to survive, they are not a necessary part of our existence now. There are a variety of other source for calcium, the main nutrient people think of when they think of dairy. These include leafy green, nuts, and tofu to name a few. It is certainly easy to take a calcium supplement if you are worried as well. High protein diets are known to leach calcium into the urine. This is why the countries with the highest calcium intakes also tend to have the highest rates of osteoporosis.

The main disadvantage of dairy products when we are trying to lose weight is the fat content. Milk is labeled based on fat per volume. One percent milk has one percent of its volume as fat but yet most of its calories from fat. That makes it very easy to drink a great number of calories in a very short time. Cheese also one of those things that is very easy to eat in excess. Its fat content, mouth feel, and savory qualities make it so you can eat multiple servings without realizing it. And most things like pizza these days by no means have one serving of cheese per single slice. Most pizza is literally dripping with cheese. Cheese is also seems to be ubiquitous these days. No longer does cheese take months of aging nor is it served in savory slivers with a cheese slicer. It is in everything as a flavoring, adding salt and fat, making it hard to stop eating all kinds of foods from snacks to main dishes. Dairy is also full of hormones. Those same hormones that make a mother and infant bond, and feel loving and relaxed, are there for the same purpose for the mothers and offspring of other mammals and are there in their whole form, or one degraded by the heating and processing of milk for human consumption. Might it be that these are the substances that make many of us classify dairy as a comfort food, slowing us down, and filling us up? If you want to lose weight, the experiences of people in this study show that the initial limiting and then elimination of dairy products of all forms can be an essential and effective component of lasting weight loss.

I am forever astounded by the number of cake-mixes and frostings available in the grocery store. Baking from scratch is nearly a lost art. Luckily in recent years though, a number of new whole grain flours have made their appearance in a limited market. Baking, from scratch, with whole grains puts you in touch with your food and is a relaxing, enjoyable, learning experience. Dumping a mix into a box, cracking an egg, and whisking is mindless, removes you from the contents, and puts a lot of needless chemicals in your body. Did you know that those mixes are engineered so that you can put largely different amounts of what they tell you add (water for instance) and they still come out right? That takes chemicals! Do yourself and your loved-ones a favor and bake using whole grains and the best ingredients. You'll bake less often, but the results will be much healthier and tastier!

And for the last subject on our quiz, cholesterol is only in foods of animal origin. If you are vegan, you never eat cholesterol. The USDA recommends getting less than 300 mg per day cholesterol in your diet.[111] While there has been less emphasis on cholesterol intake lately than on saturated fat in regard to heart disease risk, high intakes of both of these substances are related to heart disease. Where the confusion comes in is concerning blood levels of cholesterol and other fatty substances. Your blood cholesterol is related to a number of things including folic acid consumption and a healthy weight, both things that most vegetarians have going for them. Vegans have the lowest total and non-HDL serum concentrations, more so than vegetarian, fish-eaters, and meat-eaters.[112] They also have tend to have the lowest BMI and the lowest intake of saturated fats.[113] So, go ahead and eat your high folic acid veggies (dark green and orange) and steer clear those animal products.

<u>Vegetarian or Vegan?</u>

Most people will say both of these ideas are radical. Vegetarians may say vegan is radical. And, yes, vegans will say, "Why doesn't she just say vegan?"

If you are a vegan, you can be an overweight or even obese vegan. I'm not here to say you can't. You may be healthier than you would be if you ate a lot of animal products, but you may still not be as healthy as you could be if you were a normal weight. I am not here to tell you that being overweight or obese is healthy on any dietary plan, because being overweight is unhealthy regardless of what you eat.

If you are vegetarian, becoming a vegan may very well help you achieve your weight loss goals, especially if you rely on eggs and dairy products. If you eat meat, you may be a healthy

---

[111]Cholesterol. FDA. https://www.accessdata.fda.gov/scripts/interactivenutritionfactslabel/cholesterol.html

[112] K E Bradbury, F L Crowe, P N Appleby, J A Schmidt, R C Travis & T J Key. Serum concentrations of cholesterol, apolipoprotein A-I and apolipoprotein B in a total of 1694 meat-eaters, fish-eaters, vegetarians and vegans. European Journal of Clinical Nutrition volume 68, pages 178–183 (2014).

[113] Ibid.

weight, but still, unknowingly, suffer from the adverse health effects that eating a diet containing animal products is bound to bring, if not now, later in life.

If you are a meat eater and overweight or obese, and you are attached to your diet, I would very much like to see you decease your consumption of all animal products. You might do this gradually, or in one fair swoop, and I really don't care what you call yourself. Any reduction in animal products is a wonderful way to lose weight and become healthier. You can become vegetarian or vegan, but by thinking about your diet in terms of these general categories, you have a better shot at long-lasting weight loss than trying to count calories, or fat grams, or percent protein, or any other such thing.

Foods that Make You Retain Water.

There are a lot of foods that make you feel bloated. A lot of people commonly think of this as water retention. Some of this may indeed be water retention, that is, food that makes you hold onto water and you can see in changes in your daily weight. Much of this water retention though is excess weight, and this excess weight is associated with inflammation. By having the cells full, or inflamed, it is believed to contribute to ongoing, chronic diseases like heart disease, arthritis, and cancer. So, whether you are inflamed because of water or fat, neither is good.

We think of salt as making us thirsty and holding onto water, but fatty, greasy foods will do the same thing. So will sugar. So, if you are feeling puffy and bloated, skip the fat, salt, and sugar. Sodium separate from table salt itself (sodium chloride) can also be found in an abundance of food additives found in processed foods. Read the sodium content of processed foods before you purchase them avoiding monosodium glutamate (MSG), baking soda, sodium nitrite, sodium saccharin, and sodium benzoate. Unfortunately, many so-called healthy vegetarian soups have an exorbitant amount of sodium. Please read the labels! I don't know why some companies think that salt is the only flavor people can taste.

Some of these instant soups I have seen have 800 mg or more sodium per serving. Is it any wonder I was dying of thirst all day and then had a migraine after I had one of these? You need to drink more to dilute the content of the sodium in your system. For some people this feels like stiffness or bloating. For me, it causes high blood pressure and migraines.

Any foods that are both vegan and high in water content can help hydrate and nourish the body. If you feel like you are retaining water and need some particular "detoxification," you might try eating some celery, watermelon, bananas, berries, cantaloupe, carrots, lemon, cucumbers, or leafy greens. You could also try dandelion, ginger, or cinnamon teas. In any event, keep trying to exercise. Moving keeps the fluids in your body circulating and pushes the fluid in your extremities back up to your heart, as does keeping good sleeping habits.

<u>High Water Foods That Help You Feel Full.</u>
Most plant-based foods are high in water content and/or high in fiber content. This combination is ideal to help you feel full and satisfied. Your stomach only contains so much space, about a quart, and by filling it with more plant foods, which are low in calories and high in nutrients, you can be more satisfied. Most all vegan foods fit the bill. Fruits and vegetables are full of fiber, low calories, and fill you up either cooked or raw. Try making some vegetable soups or stews. They are both high water content and high in nutrients. They can also be comforting. They are warm and you can eat a lot without feeling guilty. Steer away from heavy milk, cream, or butter bases, and from beef or chicken stocks. Non-health-aware chefs say that they add flavor and mouth-feel, but they really just add fat and salt.

To make a vegetable soup, start with a little extra virgin olive oil in a big stock pot. Sauté your choice of onions, celery, and/or carrots until just browned. Any other vegetable that you want to get a little browned are also good to add at this stage. Try shallots, scallions, leeks, or fennel. This is also a good stage to add some spices, especially pepper (always a good addition to a hearty soup). When just browned but not all the way cooked, fill you pot with good quality water. I always use filtered water. Any liquid that you cook with will always become more concentrated, so make sure your water is what you would normally, happily drink. If the water in your neighborhood is normally heavily chlorinated, it is going to lend that flavor to your cooking. I know sometimes it can just smell like a swimming pool coming out of the tap. Using good, quality water is just like using any other ingredients when you cook: Use the best quality you can. After filling you pot with water, bring it to a boil and then add your choice of dried or canned beans, or cooked or uncooked grain. The hardness and size of these will change your cooking time. For a quick soup, add drained, canned beans or a leftover, cooked grain (like rice). For a soup that you can let cook a couple hours, use a big, dry bean like navy beans or limas. As you cook, occasionally stir your pot making sure you have enough water and that you have the temperature high enough to generate a simmer, but not so high that it burns, overflows, or cooks the living daylights out of your vegetables. Toward the end of cooking you can add any other vegetables that just need to soften-up like parsley and add a little dash of whatever spices you might like to adjust. A big pot of soup is a comfort to keep on hand in the refrigerator to heat up in a wink when you are hungry and really want to eat in a snap.

<u>The Negative Effects of Yo-Yo Dieting.</u>
It doesn't matter what kind of diet you do to lose weight. On every diet, as long as you cut calories, you will lose eight to fifteen pounds, maybe if you are lucky twenty. Those people that are on television advertisements about how great this or that diet is and how they lost fifty to one hundred pounds are what researchers call outliers. That is, they are the exception, not the rule. They are the odd balls. If you look at real research papers, it doesn't matter what the diet is, people usually lose less than twenty pounds.

The other thing those ads don't tell you is how long those

people took to lose that weight. It could have taken them years and years. They could have gone on and off the program for months or years at a time. Those food delivery programs cost $250.00 and up a month, plus you also have to add foods to the program, like produce and dairy, which adds to the cost.

Those food delivery programs also create tremendous waste. Every meal you get is prepackaged in both recyclable and non-recyclable plastic.

Nutrisystem reported revenue of $194.9 million for the second *quarter* of 2017.[114] Think of all those people generating waste. The majority of those people are getting monthly packaged, frozen meals shipped in huge rectangular Styrofoam containers that are not recyclable and will barely fit in a garbage can. I'm guessing now, but they're maybe two and half feet by two feet by one and a half feet. They are big. Think of all that waste in landfills.

Now Nutrisystem's price per month is about $250.00. That is $3000.00 per year for the cost of food just from them plus what you have to buy on your own. Average food cost per year for a family of four is $6,602 for the whole family for everything they eat.[115] Almost half the money you spend on food would be going to Nutrisystem. They really want you to go on the program with your spouse, too. Then you also have to worry about what everyone else is going to eat as well. You can make separate meals for the other members of the family, breakfast, lunch, and dinner, or you can buy convenience food for them, too, which adds to your overall cost as well. Yes, Nutrisystem and the other products like them are convenience food. They are not health food. They are little servings of precooked, highly processed, cheaply produced, prepackaged, chemical laden food.

---

[114] Nutrisystem Announces Second Quarter 2017 Financial Results, Exceeding Expectations. Nutrisystem, July 26th, 2017. https://newsroom.nutrisystem.com/nutrisystem-announces-second-quarter-2017-financial-results-exceeding-expectations/
[115] Average Household Cost of Food. Value Penguin. Figures for 2013. https://www.valuepenguin.com/how-much-we-spend-food

So, what do programs like Nutrisystem teach you to do? Number one, they teach you to eat low bulk. This is exactly what you do not want to do and is a very poor strategy for long term weight loss and maintenance. You can eat very small portions of their meals: their mini-muffins, tiny bagels, and fractions of a cup of soup, but very low bulk diets are difficult to sustain. Unless you are filling up with lots of vegetables on the side, you are not going to get full. That lack of fullness, that lack of satiety, is difficult to sustain in the long run. Being able to feel full helps us actually eat less overall. We yell at our kids, we are grumpy, we can't concentrate, we fight with our spouse, and whatever else when we are hungry. A sustainable diet satisfies. The diet is this book is sustainable. The proof is in all of those trim healthy vegetarians and vegans out there. (Pardon me for saying both so many times. While I advocate a vegan diet, the truth in that most of the research studies out there are on vegetarians. This is probably because there are many more vegetarians to study and because they belong to certain other groups, such as the Seventh Day Adventists, which make them easier for researchers to track down and study. Mind you, the closer you get to a vegan diet, the healthier, and slimmer, you may be.)

The human stomach is about the size of a quart container. You know, like a quart of milk. You can only put so much in it at a time. We will talk about this more latter, but for now know that we tend to eat the same volume of food day after day. Picture it. Think of that tiny portion of weight-loss food in that quart-sized container. Is that pre-packaged meal going to keep anyone happy very long? I know it won't work long for me.

This is the exact reason that people go on and off programs like Nutrisystem. You are initially motivated, so the program works, just like any new, novel program would. Then you get sick of it. You can't stand the hunger. You can't stand the monotony of the meals, even if they give you a big choice. You get sick of not being able to eat out, or heating up your little meals at work, or being finished in just a few bites, your kids and husband needing their food made, and the kids asking to try your "special" food, too.

So, you go off the program. What then? Well, these diet programs did not teach you how to eat. If you saved the containers the food came in, then maybe you can use them a guide for "potion control." But honestly, most people wouldn't even think of this.

People can't cook how Nutrisystem and similar companies manufacture their foods. You wouldn't want to either. They lack fiber and are full of sodium just to start. Maybe if you're sensitive like some people this caused you to be constipated, or feel puffy, or even have headaches or migraines as a result. This doesn't even consider the multitudes of chemicals and highly processed "foods" that are added to these so-called "healthy" foods.

The bigger you are the more calories you need. That is, the bigger you are, the more your caloric requirement will differ from one of those pre-packaged meal programs. "You eat the food; you lose the weight." Yeah, but that is pretty much the only food you can eat and you will only lose weight as long as your specific caloric requirement is more than the amount they provide, and as long as you can control yourself not to eat more than what they say you can. Now this may sound simple enough, but what these companies don't tell you is that many of the so-called "foods" in their products will actually cause you to crave not just more food, but certain specific foods as well. That is, your so called "lack of will power" to which so many overweight people feel guilty about, and so many average weight people criticize them about, may in actuality be caused by certain "foods" triggering the brain to make you want to eat. More on the specifics of this later, but for now know that anything that you have to work on, on a day-to-day basis, anything that you have to think about and actively fight against, will eventually be a losing battle, and you will give in when you are tired, or stressed, or whatever, especially when there are specific chemicals in your brain that are being triggered for you to fight against. In other words, your biology is telling you to eat, and you can only fight it so long. Why would you want to eat a food that made you want to do anything like that? If you feel the same way I do, stay away from all those packaged, pre-processed factory foods loaded with fat, sugar, salt, and animal by-products.

So, people go off the diet. They attribute it to boredom or emotional weakness or whatever. They don't know how or what to eat, because their pre-packaged food or drink mix diet didn't teach them how or what to eat. Then guess what happens? They gain the weight back. Then guess what happens next. They go back on Nutrisystem or onto the next "diet du jour." The companies count on this. If you have ever been on any of these programs you know that they will target you with mail and email until eventually you have gained so much weight and think that you are so stupid and weak that you start paying again to get their product.

In addition, if you are on the lighter side, you can only lose so much weight on these programs. That is because they are too many calories for your stature and frame, so they will never work for you.

Commercial weight-loss diet plans have also been shown to be low in macronutrients including calcium, vitamin D, and vitamin B_{12}.[116] Maybe this is part of the reason you get sick of them, too?

So here is the dilemma: Go on and off the program weight cycling or stay on the program forever? How much money do you really want to spend? And how much hardship do you really want to have to feel fighting hunger?

Weight cycling, yo-yoing up and down, is detrimental to your health. It is associated with total increased mortality, especially mortality due to cardiovascular problems.[117] Weight cycling may change body fat distribution increasing abdominal

---

[116] G Engel M, J Kern H, Brenna JT, H Mitmesser S. Micronutrient Gaps in Three Commercial Weight-Loss Diet Plans. Nutrients. 2018 Jan 20;10(1).

[117] R W Jeffery. Does weight cycling present a health risk? The American Journal of Clinical Nutrition, Volume 63, Issue 3, March 1996, Pages 452S–455S.

obesity and the associated cardiovascular risk.[118] And the longer you stay at a certain weight, the greater the chance you will continue to stay at that weight.

Do you have to stay on a diet of one sort or another forever? No, I tell you. However, some foods may not be suitable for you.

You say, "That is not fair!"

My response to that is, "It is a wonderful thing to know which foods your body responds to in a negative way!"

Most everyone eats foods that are bad for them. The problem in not knowing what foods are bad for you is that the older you are when you do find out what is bad for you, the harder it is to undo the damage.

Think of it this way. It is like the sixty-year old man who goes outside to have a cigar. He thinks to himself, "I enjoy it. I'm sixty and in good health. Why quit now?"

Well you know the answer. Like any good child or grandchild, you would tell this man who you love: "It may not be making you sick now, but it eventually will. We love you. Please stop smoking."

It is the same thing with food.

Those foods that make you overweight or obese are the same foods that will catch-up with you later in life, if they haven't already, and make you sick. If you are overweight or obese, your risk is higher than it maybe if you weren't. But this way you have a chance to see that your body is telling you something is wrong, unlike the thin person who eats the same foods that you do and gets up one morning and has a heart attack.

If you are overweight, your body is telling you that there is something wrong. Eating animal products may be at the root of the problem.

It's time for a diet that works.

What would you say if I told you could eat a bountiful array

---

[118] Rodin J, Radke-Sharpe N, Rebuffé-Scrive M, Greenwood MR Weight cycling and fat distribution. International Journal of Obesity [01 Apr 1990, 14(4):303-310].

of foods, be healthier, feel better, have less risk for heart attack, cancer, and diabetes, live longer, and not go hungry all while achieving a healthy weight? What if that same diet made you look younger, too? What if you could have fun cooking and exploring new foods, and eat out at great restaurants and not feel deprived? What if you could make the planet a cleaner place for your children and grandchildren at the same time, decreasing pollution in both the air and water? And what if you could keep the weight off for good?

"Too good to be true," you say? No! That is exactly what a vegan diet is all about. In Chapter 7, I'm going to tell you some of the over one hundred stories from people who lost weight following this diet and kept it off. Many lost a few pounds. Some were happily surprised they lost weight when they changed their diet although this was not their original intent. Some lost a hundred pounds or more. All this and keeping it off, too! No more yo-yo diets and packaged meals and powdered drinks for you!

Over ten years ago, I asked people to tell me their weight loss stories and then I asked them to tell me how they were doing. Yes, the diet works, and people are happy and healthy as ever.

In a few simple steps, you can do it, too! Keep on your path to reducing animal products and work toward a healthy vegan diet.

CHAPTER 5

REFINING YOUR DIET

SUMMARY

- Remember that you are the sum-total of everyday, so making small changes and doing them every day can make a big difference.
- What you were taught about food as a child was not necessarily correct and does not have to be how you think about it now.
- You don't have to define your diet by other people's standards. Experiment and find the foods and eating pattern that work best for you.

6 MORE THINGS TO TRY ON YOUR ROAD TO WEIGHT LOSS

I lost 65 pounds in the past nine months by becoming a vegetarian and doing light exercise (walking and jogging). My wife made the change with me and she lost 20 pounds, too!

More Ideas.

So much has been written on the subject of weight loss. Not all of it works. Much of it is fads and much of it is not based in science. Here are some more things that I find may help, plus a little inspiration.

More Measurements.

Do you like taking measurements? Here are some to try. Use a string or a cloth measuring tape. Take your measurements and re-measure every so often to keep yourself motivated and track your progress. Sometimes tracking your weight can be discouraging, and you may see more progress on your measurements. Try taking your measurements about once a month.

Most of these are self-explanatory but scientists have specific ways of doing them. For your records just be sure to measure at the same spot the same way for consistency's sake.

Ladies: Measure your bust. Measure all the way around your bust and your back on a level line. Write your measurement here:
Bust measurement: _______________________

Men and women measure your chest. (Ladies measure your chest by measuring around your chest underneath your breasts.)
Chest measurement: _______________________

Measure your waist at its narrowest point.
Waist measurement: _______________________

Measure your hips at the widest point.
Hip measurement: _______________________

Measure the widest part of your thighs.
Thigh measurement: _______________________

Measure your knees just above the knee.
Knee measurement: _______________________

Measure the calves around the fullest part.
Calf measurement: _______________________

Measure your upper arm above the elbow at the fullest part.
Upper arm measurement: _______________________

Measure your forearms below the elbows at the fullest point.
Lower arm measurement: _______________________

Hear is another fun one: Hip to waist ratio. Take your measurement for your waist and divide it by the measurement for your hip circumference. Most men think women are most attractive with a hip to waist ratio of 0.7 is most attractive. It doesn't matter what your weight is for this. You can be sexy at many different weights and body types. The hip to waist ratio relates to your ability to reproduce. Men see this as sexy since it probably relates to being more fertile.

Hip to Waist ratio = hip measurement / waste measurement
= ________________

Here is a chart for keeping track of your most important measurements.

Personal Measurement Record:

Date				
Weight				
Neck Circumference				
Bust and/or Chest Circumference				
Waist Circumference				
Hip Circumference				
Sagittal Abdominal Height (stomach height in inches when laying down)				
Thigh Circumference				
Knee Circumference				
Calf Circumference				
Upper arm Circumference				
Lower arm Circumference				

How Healthy Are the Innuits?

The Innuits are often cited as the reason to have a high protein diet. But, did you know that the Innuits live on ice flows half of the year and their water source is ice, that is, partially desalinated water? The ice on ice flows is sea water and we all know that the ocean in salty. The freezing process only slightly lowers this salt content. Much of their food consists of soups made with this brackish water. They also add caribou blood to their soups. This blood is also a rich source of sodium. High protein diets can lead to electrolyte imbalances due to uncompensated sodium loss and increased potassium excretion. This can lead to cardiac arrhythmias and muscle wasting. The Innuits have a high sodium intake.

One of the principle components of the Macrobiotic diet, which has been highly beneficial in the treatment of many cancers, is that we should eat local foods in season. Boy oh boy, that sounds like shop local; eat local. The healthiest diets may very well be the ones grown close to where we live. Now unless you are an Inuit living in the Artic, you probably shouldn't be eating the way they do. The Innuits live on a very low carbohydrate diet with brackish water and caribou blood, a high protein, high sodium diet. They also have terrible bones with very high rates of osteoporosis. Remember, excess protein causes calcium to be leached from your bones. Should we all be eating (drinking) caribou blood? Maybe someone is going to import it. I don't think that one is going to catch on! I do see "bone broth" for sale though in the so-called "health food" section. I don't think that is a very good idea either.

Nutritional ketosis, that is weight loss on a high protein low carbohydrate diet, needs medical supervision. You should have a complete medical history and physical before starting. This should include complete blood counts, thyroid test, an electrocardiogram, glycosylated hemoglobin, c-peptide, c-reactive protein, Vitamin D, hormone evaluation, screening for polycystic ovarian syndrome, urinary analysis, and a glucose tolerance test.[119] You should also have a follow-up physical and blood tests including electrolytes, renal function, liver function, fasting lipid profile, thyroid function, and other blood tests. Any abnormal blood values need to be repeated. Muscle cramps may occur, and potassium and should thus be evaluated.[120] Certain nutrients are difficult to maintain without some fruits and vegetables. Also, if you are already taking any medications, you can also run into problems which require medical supervision. To me, weaning yourself off animal products sounds a whole lot easier than all of this hoopla in going almost exclusively animal protein and fat.

Noah's Ark.
Did you know that the diet on Noah's Arc was vegetarian? All of the animals and humans lived in peace. What a wonderful thing to aspire to!

Fish is not a Vegetable.
Don't other people say fish is good for you? Well, some people say that certain kinds of fish are good for you for the omega-3 fatty acid content in the prevention of heart disease. But veganism is probably the best thing you can do for the prevention of heart disease. Because a vegan diet is low in saturated fatty acids and higher in monounsaturated and polyunsaturated fatty acids, it aids in the prevention of heart disease. Omega-3 fatty acids are found in certain fish, but they are also high in nuts and seeds, their oils, and fortified foods. This includes flax, walnuts, chia, soy, hemp, canola oil, as well as seaweeds like nori and algae, kidney beans, broccoli, basil, spinach, cashews, and Brussel sprouts. They are especially high in flax oil. If you like, you can take a flax oil supplement. Flax oil is also a fine oil to top your salad, toast, or cooked vegetables with. It is on the thin side, so it doesn't have much mouth feel. It also has only a slight taste. It is not strong;

---

[119] Steelman, G. Michael (Editor), Westman, Eric C. (Editor)Obesity: Evaluation and Treatment Essentials, Second Edition 2nd Edition. CRC Press, New York, 2016.
[120] Ibid.

people always say it is a little nutty. I like flax oil on my salad or cooked squash with a grind of pepper and some mixed, salt-free herb blend (like Italian or dried vegetable flakes).

Fish contains all kinds of toxins that are found in our unfortunately polluted oceans. Fish that are farmed are not eating the natural things that they would in the wild. Farmed salmon is fed dye to make its fresh the natural pink, orange color that we think of as salmon. Farmed salmon would be gray in color without it. Like other animal products, fish can be full of chemicals. And while we may not think of fish as being particularly cute or cuddly, their skin/scales are extremely sensitive. Just holding them can remove the protective layer of mucus on them so much that they can get infections and die if you pick them up and throw them back in. Anyway, eating fish is not necessary. My father once almost died by having a fish bone caught in his throat – yet something else you won't have to worry about.

This is Not a Diet; This is a Lifestyle.

When you transition to a vegetarian and then vegan diet, you could do it all at once or you could do it gradually. One thing is clear though from my research, those who when on and off the diet had their weight yo-yo up and down. This yo-yoing in very bad for your overall health, especially your heart, no matter what diet you are on. You should not think that becoming a vegetarian or a vegan is a bad thing, an act of deprivation. Think of the foods you are eliminating as a bad thing that aren't good for you, that is, for you as an individual. You don't have to be militant and tell everyone that meat is bad for them, too, although it very well may be.

Those participants who lost weight when they became vegetarian, lost more weight when they became vegan, but gained it back again when they added animal products back into their diets. Those who stayed at the vegan level, or whatever level they wanted to maintain, maintained their weight loss, which we know is much more difficult, and therefore impressive.

<u>Think About It this Way.</u>

Not all foods are good for all people. Think of this. If you were allergic to a particular food and had a horrible reaction to it, you may want to avoid it for life. You would know that it just wasn't good for you. It wouldn't matter to you how many people around the world ate that food every single day, to you it would be poison. By eliminating any particular food, we can tell our own particular body's reaction to it. If we eliminate it from our diet for a long enough time, we may see weight loss or even weight gain depending on exactly what it did to the body. By eliminating animal products, we know from studies that it is possible to lose weight. It does not even really matter what the reason is for this reaction. It could be decreasing the fat in the diet, the total calories in the diet, decreasing added chemicals, increasing fiber, increasing satiety, changing the rate of digestion, decreasing the caloric density, increasing the volume of food, changing the neurologic response to food, altering our hormone levels, or whatever. It doesn't really matter how it works. If a diet is health, and it works for you, you are the boss. You can eat what you want and see how your body responds.

You can also reintroduce any given food and see how your body responds, as many of my respondents did. Seeing how your body responds when you reintroduce any non-vegan or non-vegetarian product can be a great learning experience. You could notice nothing. But you could feel lousy the next day, as some people report (e.g. headaches, feeling bloated, achy joints etc.) You could also notice weight gain. If you notice any adverse reaction, this can be a real learning experience and reinforcer.

My father had a very definite experience like this. When I was a teenager, I was at a vegetarian conference and met Dr. Michael Klapper. Now Dr. Klapper is a very sweet, patient man. My father at the time was having some very unusual reactions and wasn't getting any answers from the doctors in our area. When my mom came and met me at the conference, she arranged for my dad to call Dr. Klapper. Well, that night

Dr. Klapper spent three hours on the telephone talking to my father. I am not exaggerating!

Now my father was a very stubborn man. He ran a factory, he was in charge, he was the boss, and consequently, he was a know-it-all. (That's okay. Aren't we all?) But my father was having strange symptoms. Every now and again, half of his face would puff up and it was getting worse. His cheek, and then his chin, his lips, his neck – and it was getting worse. Now Dr. Klapper was convinced that is was an allergy to "too much foreign protein" in his system. My father ate a lot of meat. In fact, if there was no meat, there was no meal. When we went out to eat, without exception, he would get the biggest, most expensive piece of meat on the menu. Remember he was the boss, and when he went out to eat he had to prove it. Dr. Klapper also told him to go to a particular allergist for specific tests.

Well, they did find specific things my father was allergic to (aspirin, sulfites- he was a big red wine drinker). My dad also became vegetarian, much to his chagrin. But my mom was becoming our own gourmet chef, and the food was really good, so he stuck with it at home. My mom would pack him a breakfast and lunch. He was happy and most importantly did not have any symptoms. Dr. Klapper had really scared him it turns out. Prior to this my father had noticed that the symptoms were getting worse. Dr. Klapper told him that they would continue to get worse to the point that his neck would eventually swell up so much that the swelling would cut off his airway and he would suffocate to death. Now, as you know, my dad was the boss, and he wanted to be the boss of his own body, too, so he gave up all meat. The thing is though, while things were fine at home, when he went out to dinner with his friends or on a business meeting, and my mother was not around, he would once again get the biggest, most expensive piece of meat on the menu. He had to show off his prowess in front of the men, right? Can you believe, every single time he did this, the next day his face would blow-up! He looked like he had been in a fight. Eventually, this happened one too many times, and he learned his lesson and gave up all meat for good.

I'm not suggesting that anything remotely like this may happen to you. My father was unique in more ways than one. You might notice specific symptoms. It is my guess, however, that your major symptom is your weight.

<u>Exercise Recommendations for Weight Maintenance.</u>
Did you know that the exercise recommendation for those who were obese and then achieved a healthy weight is a whopping 60 to 90 minutes a day? And that is actual exercise, not just physical activity. When we think of exercise recommendations, we always think of that recommendation of 30 minutes a day for most days of the week. But what people don't realize is that this recommendation is for health maintenance for people who have never been obese/overweight. This recommendation is not for weight loss. And it certainly isn't for those who were obese! 60 to 90 minutes is the recommendation for those who were obese and lost weight. This is because the body has been preconditioned to storing fat at the same level it did when that individual was obese.

Try this for an exercise. Think of how much weight you want to lose. Find something that weighs about that amount or less and try carrying it around with you for as much of the day as you can. If you don't have much to lose, you could try carrying a weight or a gallon of water. A gallon of water weighs 8.34 pounds. So if you want to lose twenty pounds, that is like carrying almost two and a half gallons of water around with you. You could try carrying weight in a back pack or in your pockets. My husband even has a weight vest. Try carrying around with you however much weight you can for as long as you are able, then put the weight down or take it off. How light do you feel? That is how light you will feel when you lose that weight. You may even want to make this part of your exercise routine. Now think about all that extra weight that you have to carry around with you everywhere you go. That weight is literally holding you down. Think how much more you will be able to do and how much better you will feel when you lose that excess weight.

As you have experienced, carrying extra weight is hard. That is why, obese people sit on average two and a half hours more per day than other people. The more you sit at any given time, the body's metabolic rate slows to something close to your metabolic rate when you are sleeping. Every if you don't have time, or can't exercise, get up and move around. The more you do during the day, the more you boost your metabolic rate.

The longest-lived people in the world generally live on mountains. They walk up and down daily, both young and old. You may not have a mountain to climb but walk up and down a bunch of stairs every day. I call the stairs in my house, "My Mountain." I can get up the stairs pretty quick carrying a basket of laundry, too. Don't worry. I've experienced weight gain, too. I have three kids, and one of my favorite jokes is:

The doctor ask a woman, "How long have you been this heavy?"

"Since I had the baby," she replies.

"How old is the baby?" he asks.

"Oh, he's ten."

Life happens. One of the best things you can do along with your vegan diet is add exercise to your routine. It is time for you and it is great for your overall health.

<u>Adding Exercise to Your Program.</u>

There are overall health benefits of exercise apart from weight loss and those who exercise while they are trying to lose weight maintain muscle. If you compare weight loss with exercise to weight loss without, in those who lost weight without exercise over thirty percent of the weight lost was from lean tissue.[121] Muscle is necessary for movement,

---

[121] Ballor DL, Poehlman ET. Exercise-training enhances fat-free mass preservation during diet-induced weight loss: a meta-analytical finding. international Journal of Obesity and Related Metabolic Disorders : Journal of the International Association for the Study of Obesity [01 Jan 1994,

strength, and health. Our immune system is tied to the amount of muscle we have and as we get older most people lose muscle anyway. Don't we want to lose fat not muscle? Then, be sure you exercise when you are on a weight loss program.

First, pick an exercise that you like to do. That means that it is something that you will actually do, not just say you will do at some indefinite time in the future.

Next, try to do something aerobic, that is, something that will move you around while consuming air. This might include walking, jogging, running, cycling, etc. If your BMI classifies you as obese (see Chapter 3), the European College of Sports Science recommends moderate-intensity exercise daily, and vigorous activity every other day.[122] Remember that the exercise intensity will depend on you, how you feel, and what you are capable of, not anyone else. Do you best and try not to compare yourself with anyone else. What you should strive to do is to compare yourself to yourself. Try to make yourself the best you can be. I am sure we have all head to keep track of how much you exercise. We could also try to keep track of the intensity of the exercise and if the exercise we do is getting easier. One way to do this is to use a heart rate monitor. A heart rate monitor is like having a personal trainer on your wrist.

Have you ever put your hands on two metal pads of a piece of electronic exercise equipment at the gym and had the machine give you your heart rate? This is a quick heart rate monitor. The old-fashioned way used to be to stop and count your pulse while looking at a clock for fifteen seconds then multiplying the number by four to get beats per minute. If you have ever tried to do this, you know it can be difficult to be accurate. You probably have to stop exercising and you often get mixed-up, because after all, you are supposed to be working out. The most accurate heart rate monitors have chest

---

18(1):35-40].
[122] Mikael Fogelholm, Bente Stallknecht, Marleen Van Baak. ECSS position statement: Exercise and obesity. European Journal of Sport Science. Volume 6, 2006 - Issue 1.

straps and a wrist watch. If you buy a good one you will be able to take it anywhere you exercise including in the water. There are also apps that will do this, but ones with the chest strap will be the most accurate.

Heart rate monitors enable you to find your best heart rate training zones for your age and fitness level. By doing this you will be able to tell such things as:

- You are working too hard and should slow down,
- You should work harder,
- You are in the optimum heart rate zone for fat loss,
- You are in an optimum endurance training zone,
- You are in an aerobic zone and using oxygen or you are in an anaerobic zone and using glycogen (as in sprinting)
- How fast you can bring your heart rate from a rapid rate to a calm rate (recovery rate)
- And a range of other features like lap times and alarms.

By using a heart rate monitor, you can track your specific goals. Interestingly enough, most people who are trying to lose weight have a tendency to go too hard. Body builders have long known that they have to do "LSD." No, I am not kidding, because LSD is Long, Slow Distance. By tracking your optimum "low" heart rate for fat burning while doing extensive periods of exercise, they know that is how to get rid of the fat. You only ever see body builders struggling lifting heavy weights or doing slow exercise on one of the cardio machines. You never see them running or cycling like crazy, sweating to death doing cardio. They know that is not the way to lose fat while preserving muscle. Running and sweating like crazy is good for other things like your heart or feeling happy. Learning about your heart rate will help your train smarter and, quite frankly, help you not overdo it, get too sore, and miss training days. We have all regretted exercising too hard on occasion. Some soreness and tiredness is good. It makes you feel alive and strengthens your bones and muscles. But going overboard, especially in the beginning can cause us to be so sore and lethargic that we can barely do anything the next day or two, and often eat way more than we know we should. By the way, if you work out very hard, be warry of delayed-onset muscle soreness. The second day after exercise is often when exercise-induce muscle soreness is the worst.

So what heart rate should you strive for? That depends on your age, fitness, exercise goals, and the purpose of that individual workout. The American Heart Association has guideline for target heart rate zones and the average maximum heart rate values.[123] Whatever method you use though to determine your exercise intensity, play it by ear. We all have our good days when it comes to exercise. What is good one day may not be good then next if you are tired, sick, or stressed to the max. Take care of yourself and if you feel like you may be overdoing it, stop.

Next, add some resistance training. Even a little bit of "weight lifting" preserves muscle which is especially important as we get older. While I don't want to be a body builder, I still want to be able to open a jar when I am an old lady, and I'm sure you want to as well. Strength training works at all ages. Even lifting cans of soup has been shown to improve strength in the elderly and is extremely helpful in the prevention of accidents in the home, especially falls. Resistance training can prevent the "normal" loss of muscle that most people experience with aging. The American College of Sports Medicine recommends:

- Do large muscle groups before small muscle group exercises (e.g. legs before arms), multiple-joint exercises before single-joint exercises (e.g. lunges before biceps), and higher-intensity before lower-intensity exercises (more difficult or intense before less difficult and intense),

---

[123] You can find more information from the American Heart Association at www.heart.org.

- For novices, that the load of weight correspond to a repetition range of an 8-12 repetition maximum. For intermediate and advanced, that the load of the weight correspond to a repetition range of 1 to 12 repetitions, with 1 to 6 repetitions for the most advanced.
- Take 3 to 5 minute rests between sets.
- Train 2 or 3 days a week if you are a novice, 3 to 4 days a week if you are intermediate, and 4 or 5 days a week if you consider yourself advanced.
- Place the main part of your training on multiple joint exercises that move the entire body not just one body part (e.g. squats more than shoulder shrugs).
- For endurance training, use higher repetitions with lighter loads.
- Apply these recommendations in context and contingent upon an your individual goals, physical capacity and health, and your training status. That is, don't overdo it but give yourself a good workout. Don't worry, ladies. You are not going to "bulk-up." That takes a lot more effort than most people are willing to put in.[124]

Remember, when it comes to diet and exercise, a body builder and a dietitian are going to give you different opinions. Even their definition of the word health may be different. A body builder may think that a dietitian is a scrawny weakling, and the dietitian may think that the body builder is a lug-head who knows nothing about nutrition. Keep researching, make-up your own mind, and find the best routine that works for you.

---

[124] American College of Sports Medicine. American College of Sports Medicine position stand. Progression models in resistance training for healthy adults. Med Sci Sports Exerc. 2009 Mar;41(3):687-708.

<u>Weight Loss as Famine.</u>
Fat (adipose tissue) is an active, hormonal tissue that fights for its survival. In an age when food was scare, which let's face it was most of our heritage, we needed these mechanisms to maintain our weight and health, by encouraging eating, gluttony, and gorging when food was available to ensure our survival.

When we try to lose weight, the body thinks that we are living through a famine, and it fights desperately to maintain our weight. This is why it is important to do two things. First, you should not try to lose weight quickly. This signifies to the body that we are sick and starved, so it will fight to gain the weight back.

Second, you really should seek to lose one pound or so a week. This represents just enough calories to cause a deficit and weight reduction, but not enough to that that body switches into panic mode.

Third, you should actively seek to eat a high nutrient density diet. This is a major contributor of a vegetarian/vegan diet to weight loss.

<u>More on the Nutrient Density of Vegan Foods.</u>
As you know, when I was growing up, the horse and donkeys would chew on the wooden fence if you didn't give them a salt lick. Not just a plain salt lick, it had to be one with minerals in it. If they didn't have it, they would literally chew through a railing. The goats would do a similar thing, but they always seemed to want the bushes, like the holly and pine, that my mother did not want them to eat.

Now studies have been done with goats (and monkeys and other animal, too), that they will seek out and eat certain foods when they are sick or lacking in a specific nutrient. I really believe we are that way, too. Here is my reasoning. The more processed foods you eat, the less of the naturally occurring vitamins, minerals, and whatever other substances are in them that we haven't defined. Remember, we can't make a carrot. Modern science thinks that they have solved the problems of processed foods by adding back key nutrients and solving all of the modern problems of deficiency diseases while keeping food from perishing. They solved the mysteries pellagra (B3/niacin), beriberi (B1/thiamine), scurvy (vitamin C), goiter (iodine), rickets (vitamin D), anemia (iron, B12, and folate), osteoporosis (calcium), and folates relation to neural tube defects. But what else does food contain? Is this it? They have eliminated many, many of the problems with the perishability of food by milling, canning, freezing, dehydrating, adding numerous chemicals, fillers, and preservatives. They have high temperature baked, fried, air puffed, sifted, and filtered. They have manufactured vitamins out of petroleum, minerals out of rock, and other "foods," dyes, and additives out of who knows what.[125]

But get a load of this. There is new evidence that the more we have fortified, the more we have become obese. Yeah, we are eating more processed foods, but some researchers are linking this specifically to niacin. They think that the fortified niacin in foods is causing people to gain weight. In fact, intravenous niacin improves the efficiency of dietary fat storage.[126] Also, high levels of all of the B vitamins are correlated with obesity and diabetes.[127] Incidentally, this increase in intake is not correlated to an increase in fruits and vegetables; it is correlated to intake from artificial sources. There are biological mechanisms at work here. "B vitamins enhance fat synthesis, excess vitamins cause insulin resistance, excess vitamins may disturb neurotransmitter metabolism, and excess vitamins may involve alterations in gene expression."[128]

---

[125] Want a fun book to read on this subject. Try <u>Twinkie, Deconstructed: My Journey to Discover How the Ingredients Found in Processed Foods Are Grown, Mined (Yes, Mined), and Manipulated into What America Eats</u> by Steve Ettlinger, 2008.

[126] Nelson RH, Vlazny D, Smailovic A, Miles JM. Intravenous niacin acutely improves the efficiency of dietary fat storage in lean and obese humans. Diabetes. 2012 Dec;61(12):3172-5.

[127] Shi-Sheng Zhou, Yiming Zhou. Excess vitamin intake: An unrecognized risk factor for obesity. World J Diabetes. 2014 Feb 15; 5(1): 1–13.

What about this though? Could it be that we are like our farm animals growing up? Do we know that we are lacking something in our diets that we just can't put a finger on that makes us want to keep eating, sometimes out of control, to make sure that we get enough of that substance? And maybe, be won't get enough of whatever it is until we eat an enormous volume of processed food because it hardly contains anything.

Now I don't know what this substance is, and frankly, I don't really care, because if and when they discover something else new, as they always do, they will strip it from its natural habitat and lock it in a cage by itself for viewing and consumption. Is any vitamin really itself if it is stripped from its natural environment? Yes, you're right. I'm not a fan of zoos and I'm not a fan of isolating nutrients and adding them back to the diet. Animals are so much nicer in their natural habitat, and so are nutrients.

So here is the good news. The more my research subjects stayed with a plant-based diet and the more they stayed away from processed foods, the more their appetites balanced, and their weight balanced at a level that was healthy, and appropriate, to them.

<u>You Don't Have to Make the Change all at Once.</u>
Some people do better making a change of any sort when they plunge into it head first. I know myself that I am not one to make any kind of dramatic change if I say, "Well, I'll let myself do it (whatever my bad habit is) just once in a while." I tend to do better getting rid of any bad habit if I do not give myself leeway. You, on the other hand, may be just the opposite. There is nothing that says change has to come all at once. Any part of adapting a healthier diet and life-style is certainly worth making whenever you do it.

Improving your diet may mean cutting out red meat. Maybe, cutting out whole milk might be a start for you. Limiting eggs might be a starting point for you. Only you know

---

[128] Ibid.

yourself best, your likes and dislikes, and what motivates you.

<u>Don't Be a Fat Vegan.</u>
You might not like to hear this, but I hate to tell you it is true: You can be a vegan and still be fat. You may be healthier than you would otherwise be if you were a big meat-eater, but those extra pounds still aren't doing your health any good. Here are some traps vegans can fall into:

- Not exercising and relying on diet to do it all. Be a good example! Be active!
- Eating too much health-food, junk food. I think you know by now that eating too much processed, packaged food can't be good. Even if the food is made of exclusively "healthy" ingredients, we may pay the price by having them be too convenient. A lot of the so-called healthy snacks are nothing but sugar in another form (e.g. dates, raisins, date sugar, organic cane syrup, etc.) Sometimes, when food is too easy to grab and eat, it is too easy to eat too much. Strive for making more of your own foods and go heavier on the vegetables. In order to judge a food, you must look the individual food, how it is used, how much it is consumed, and the individual consuming it. Some health foods, vegetarian or vegan or not, are really just junk. Just because something is vegan does not mean it is heathy. You can be a junk food vegan, e.g. cola and potato chips, but you probably wouldn't feel too great. Each food should be judged on its individual merits and demerits. Something that is vegan but is loaded with sugar is going to make you feel terrible when it makes your blood sugar crash. Something that is high in sodium, like a canned soup, an instant soup cup, or pretzels, is going to make you want to eat more, number one, because it overstimulates the appetite with a high amount of salt, and number two, it is going to make you want to drink a lot. Drinking a

lot can cause you to consume too many calories (depending on what you drink and how much), cause you to consume chemicals (a diet version), and increase your blood pressure (especially if you are sensitive to such things – which I feel most people are to some degree or another).

- Eating too many "Halo Effect" foods. Some of these health-food aisle foods are health food junk foods, that is, so-called healthy foods loaded with sugar and/or fat and/or salt. Other so-called healthy foods are what they call "halo effect" foods, that is they contain one healthy item, like oat bran, or one "superfood" like whole grains, or one "super nutrient," like omega-3, and the rest of the product is given a pass and can be as unhealthy as need be in order to sell the product. Classic examples are those "healthy" sugary, vitamin cereals "made with" whole grain that just have a dose of vitamins and a dash of whole grain while the rest is highly processed white grain and sugar. Also, don't get into the habit that because you eat one "superfood" it cancels out all the other unhealthy foods (or habits) you consume. One green juice drink will not undo a doughnut. Some pomegranate juice is not going to undo a night's drinking. Pick each food for their own merits. Consider their benefits and consequences. Consider if they are fit to go into your body. You are the master of your diet. You are the boss.

- Eating too many nuts. We have all heard the news about nuts being good for us. The consumption of nuts has be associated with less heart disease, gallstones, hypertension, cancer, inflammation, lower cholesterol, weight in the midsection, and metabolic syndrome.[129] That doesn't mean we can't eat them to

---

[129] Emilio Ros. Health Benefits of Nut Consumption. Nutrients. 2010 Jul;2(7):652-82. doi: 10.3390/nu2070683. Epub 2010 Jun 24.

excess though. They are one of those natural convenience foods that we can easily overdo. Try limiting yourself to about an ounce a day. That is just a handful. Try measuring that amount. A shot glass is a handy tool. A shot glass is an ounce and a half, so don't fill it up all the way. Two tablespoons is also an ounce. Now I know this is fluid ounces as compared to weight, but it is a good, everyday approximation. Try measuring what you plan to eat and then putting the rest away and getting out of the kitchen. I know it can be easy to eat a jar of peanuts while watching television at night, but that isn't going to be doing you any good. Try measuring your servings. Make your serving spoon a measure.

- Eating too many grains. Grains are the staff of life, but again they can be a way of eating too many calories. Try eating more vegetables and have grains one the side or mixed with them in a smaller proportion. Also, skip the boxed cereals. Most boxed cereals are extremely highly processed. The grains are cooked to a mush and forced at ultra-high heat through and extruder and flash dried. It does not matter how many added nutrients and whatever other "healthy" ingredients they add back into these products. They cannot make them healthy to my standards. Here's why. They are processed at such unnaturally high heat that they take absolutely nothing for the body to digest. Normal, whole foods require chewing first off. These cereals essentially dissolve in milk. The manufactures are constantly trying to add chemicals, alter the processing, and especially add sugar as a coating to make a barrier to keep the milk from making them soggy. They are constantly experimenting on how to keep these foods crispy and crunchy. These factors also make you want to eat more. Sugar makes you crave more. The leftover milk in the bowl makes you want to add more cereal, so you don't waste the milk. The fun boxes beg for attention and make a distraction. Since they are so highly processed, once they get to your stomach, they simply don't need much in the way of digestion. They are already a mush with little need of churning. This means that they do not increase your body temperature when they are digested nearly as much as an unprocessed grain would. We call this increase in temperature the thermic effect of food. This increase in temperature uses energy. Unprocessed grains would also stay in the stomach longer digesting and signaling to our brains that our stomachs are full. Processed cereals essentially can skip the stomach and head to the small intestine to start to be absorbed, thus making room for more food to fill up our stomachs.

A Word on "Fake Meats."

One thing that participants in this study do not report is eating a lot of "fake meat." A lot of vegetarians, and people in general, wonder why a vegetarian would want to eat something that looked or tasted like "the original."

Let me tell you a story. Once upon a time, there was very little soy milk on the market. It used to be only available as a powder that you mixed yourself. When aseptic packaging was introduced, soy milk could be put on the health food store shelf and it really contained very few, very simple ingredients. Then "marketing genius" brought us Silk. Now Silk was pretty much like the other soy milks, maybe a little less nutritious since it had sugar and did not want to cater to the small health food segment. Silk was aseptically packed and could sit on the health food store shelf for months and months just like all the others. But what if they put a "fake milk," that did not need refrigeration in the refrigerator case next to the "real" milk? This way consumers would see it when they went to buy their milk and would view it as not just the equivalent to milk, but a healthier option.

My point is: A lot of this is marketing. We don't need fake

meats, nor highly processed milks. People in the study did not report: "Oh, I stopped eating fried chicken and started eating frozen fake "chicken nuggets." They ate whole natural foods like beans, legumes, whole grains, and the relatively low processed tofu.

"Fake meats" are about getting people interested in a new food and marketing. I am not saying these foods are unhealthy. Like any other food you must look at the individual food, how it is used, how much it is consumed, and the individual consuming it.

"Fake meats" serve as a gateway to trying vegetarian products and easing people into new tastes. That is why soy and other milks, and now even fake meats, are being placed next to their "real" counterparts to increase sales. But I am sure you realize that they are highly processed and sometimes even border the realm of junk food.

A Serious Note on Binge Eating Disorder.

Binge eating disorder is defined by the American Psychiatric Association as recurrent and persistent episodes of binge eating. Binge eating episodes are associated with three (or more) of the following: (1) Eating much more rapidly than normal, (2) Eating until feeling uncomfortably full, (3) Eating large amounts of food when not feeling physically hungry, (4) Eating alone because of being embarrassed by how much one is eating, or (5) Feeling disgusted with oneself, depressed, or very guilty after overeating, as well as marked distress regarding binge eating and the absence of regular compensatory behaviors (such as purging that would be associated with bulimia).[130] Binge eating disorder is associated with obesity and many medical conditions including type 2 diabetes, high blood pressure, high cholesterol, coronary heart disease, congestive heart failure, angina pectoris, stroke, asthma, osteoarthritis, musculoskeletal disorders, gallbladder disease, sleep apnea and

---

[130] American Psychiatric Association. Diagnostic and Statistical Manual of Mental Disorders (DSM-5®), Fifth Edition. American Psychiatric Association. Washington, D.C. 2013.

respiratory problems, gout, bladder control problems, problems with female reproductive health, and cancers of the uterus, breast, prostate, kidney, liver, pancreas, esophagus, colon, and rectum.[131] Binge eating disorder is also associated with depression, anxiety, and personality disorders such as sleep disorders and substance abuse.[132] Negative body image and weight fluctuations are also more severe with binge eating disorder.[133]

People who gravitate toward highly restrictive diets can have a tendency toward binging. If you find yourself with any of the symptoms mentioned above, know that binge eating disorder is serious and the treatments for you will be different than simple weight management alone. Research supports that mindfulness-based cognitive behavioral therapy (MBCBT) can be very effective for people like you. Since binge eating disorder is associated with stress, trauma, and the like, MBCBT can be very effective at helping you to be aware of your feelings without giving in to them.[134] While I do not think that a vegan diet is highly restrictive, but instead varied and delicious, other people might. If you find that you binge, take a good hard look at yourself. Now that you know the characteristics and the consequences of binge eating disorder, you can take steps with your health care provider to address it and overcome the weight problems and mental stresses that are associated with it. Further information is beyond the scope of this book, but can be found through the National Eating Disorders Association at www.nationaleatingdisorders.org.

<u>Understanding Obesogens.</u>
The world is full of chemicals and we all know that many of these can be harmful to human. Did you know though that

---

[131] Carson, Ralph. Binge eating disorder: Etiology, assessment, diagnosis, and treatment. Obesity: Evaluation and Treatment, Second Edition.
Steelman, G. Michael, Westman, Eric C. CRC Press, New York, 2016.
[132] Ibid.
[133] Ibid.
[134] Ibid.

certain chemicals can actual make you fat? These chemicals are called obesogens, that is they are chemicals that promote obesity. They may do this by changing the function of hormones and therefore can also be endocrine disruptors. While certain foods may cause you to eat more, certain chemicals in your environment can also have negative effects on your health, including weight gain. Any time a chemical disrupts endocrine function it can change the natural, normal function of hormones and cause great change in your health including loss of fertility. These tiny little chemicals can cause huge problems.

The good new though is the more natural you become in your diet and your lifestyle when it comes to chemical exposure, the more you can do to rid yourself of endocrine disrupting chemicals' harmful effects. Here are some simple things to do to help get these fat-promoting chemicals out of your life:

- Stop smoking in all forms. Smoking is not healthy or natural in any form. Don't kid yourself. Breathing small particulates into your lungs is a recipe for getting them trapped there with no way to get out. When a foreign body gets trapped in your body, it causes irritation and inflammation. This can be a recipe for cancer and other diseases.

- Stay away from air pollution. Try to limit your exposure to chemicals in the air in all form. This includes barbeques, campfires, lawn mowers, bus exhaust, saw dust, household dust, aerosol sprays, air fresheners, incense, and other burning or chemicals.

- Limit your exposure to flame retardants. Many of these products have proven harmful and have been taken off the market due to health concerns. Limit exposure to them the best you can. They may be found in childhood pajamas, household soft furnishings such as carpets, blinds, and items that contain foam, building materials, electronic devices, and auto parts. Washing you hands before eating or touching your face is always a good idea since we often cannot control where these products may be found.

- Limit your exposure to phthalates. These are chemicals used to soften plastics and help dissolve certain chemicals. They can make plastic more transparent, flexible, and durable. They are used in the manufacture of PVC pipe, garden hoses, pool liners, waterproof fabric, and luggage. However, they are also found in hair spray, nail polish, shampoo, makeup, perfume, laundry detergent, and other things that have fragrance. Look for natural phthalate-free products, get rid of toys and other plastics made before 2009 that may contain them, avoid plastics in the kitchen, and by all means, never cook with or heat food in plastics. These harmful chemicals will get into the food especially if they are heated. Fats tend to absorb them more.

- Avoid BPA, bisphenol A and all the other ones, too. Everything seems to be labelled BPA-free these days, but just because there is no BPA doesn't mean we are in the clear. Potentially harmful chemicals, including other bisphenols may be present. There just isn't enough information against them yet to get the public worried, and thus get them banned or labelled. BPA can also be in the lining of cans, so here is yet another reason to look for fresh foods. Try using foods packaged in glass, and again, don't heat food in plastic. Even if you by microwaveable frozen food, do your future self a favor and heat the frozen food on a glass or ceramic dish instead.

- Reduce your pesticide exposure. Pesticides are meant to affect the nervous system or other major systems of pest organisms to kill them. We are not so different from other organisms that we should not expect them to affect us. You know the deal: Buy organically produced products whenever you can and keep chemicals out of your yard and home.

<u>Easy Plan for Losing Weight: Devising a Program</u>
Remember, in order to lose weight, you must have either caloric reduction or increased caloric expenditure. All of those other magical methods for weight loss are all hoopla. There are approximately 3500 calories in a pound of fat. That is a lot, so it is going to take a lot of effort. Follow these steps to make it as easy as possible, and remember, you are in it for the long haul. Stick to it and don't give up the ship!

Step One: <u>Become a vegetarian!</u> This is the single most important thing that you can do to put yourself on the path to a healthier diet. The more meats you ate, the more effect you should see. Don't make the mistake of cutting out so-called "red meats" and replacing them with chicken and fish. It is much easier, and effective to cut them all out. You can do this all at once or step by step, but there is no reason you need them.

Step Two: <u>Become a vegan!</u> Don't make the mistake of becoming a vegetarian and replacing the meats with tons of eggs and dairy. Eggs and dairy are packed with calories, even the low-fat versions. Eggy, cheesy casseroles and pizza are by no means healthy. Again, the more you eat of them, the more you may notice when you cut them out. And don't make the mistake of replacing "real" eggs and dairy with "fake" versions. Many of the fake cheeses, etc. are packed with fat and calories. If you want to use them on occasion, that is fine, but don't make them a huge part of your diet.

Step Three: <u>Eat lots of vegetables!</u> Being a vegetarian should mean eating lots of vegetables. That is what it is supposed to mean. Vegetables should be the single most nutrient rich part of your diet. They are filling, full of fiber, packed with the most nutrients per calorie, low in calories, and the only source of life-giving phytonutrients (those nutrients found only in plants that modern, scientific research is linking to long life and disease prevention and treatment). Don't make the mistake of becoming one of those vegetarians that never eats vegetables. Eat your veggies!

Step Four: <u>Do away with as many processed foods as possible!</u> Don't be a health food, junk food junkie. Most everything that is pre-packaged is full of fat, sugar, salt, and/or other flavor enhancing chemicals that make you not only want to eat more, but for some of us unable to resist even being able to stop eating. If these products didn't have these things in them, they not only wouldn't sell to the general public, but they would not be profitable. These ingredients are cheap fillers, not quality ingredients. Healthy foods are not supposed to last on the shelf forever. You went this far to make yourself healthier. Take the next step and give up all those easy to grab "bars" in your snack drawer. They have been sitting there forever and can sit in their static form forever. They are too easy to grab and scarf down, and not nearly satisfying enough.

Step Five: <u>Pay attention to the serving size of your more concentrated foods</u>. Whole grains are great and very healthy, just don't eat unlimited quantities of them. The same goes for fruits, especially dried fruit and juice, nuts, seed, legumes, beans, tofu, etc. When you first become a vegetarian, you may not want to be so strict with yourself, but remember, there are fat vegetarians. Eating health-food junk-food and too large a portion may be their biggest trouble.

A serving size of bread is one slice, of breakfast cereal is one cup, and of cooked grains like oatmeal, rice, millet, pasta, etc. is only a half cup. So, if you eat a sandwich, you are eating two serving of bread if you eat two slices. A big bowl of pasta might even be four or more servings.

Here is an idea: When making any grain that you have to serve, dish out, or pour out, use a measuring cup or a half cup measure as your serving spoon/utensil. Taking a portion with a regular serving spoon can be deceptive. You spoon it out, it falls on your plate and spreads out, it looks good, so you take more. By using a measure, you know how much a serving is without having to guess and without having to reason with yourself that it looks good, and is healthy, so you should be fine taking a little more.

Humans are very good at keeping their daily caloric intake relatively stable. This means that when you are on a weight loss program you have to do one of two things: One, change your diet so radically that you don't know the difference, which is what eliminating animal products does, or two, change the amount of calories by so little that you do not feel that it is suffering. Most people will feel hardship with a caloric deprivation of just 200 calories a day. Any more than this is hard to maintain for any length of time. That means that you have to be patient though. 3500 calories in a pound of fat is going to take a long time to whittle away at with just a 200-calorie deprivation a day. This is why, while paying attentions to not eating in excess (that is, your serving size), making a radical change eliminating animal products is a great way to go. By changing things so completely, you are breaking away from all old habits and consciously creating new, healthier ones. But again, you're not a wolf. Don't gorge.

Step Six: <u>Don't be lazy!</u> But try not to only be a weekend warrior either. We all know that being active is good for us, but binging on exercise is a thing, too. Too much of a good thing (exercise) can leave you so sore that it makes you much less active in the days that follow. It can also make you eat too much, that is, consume more calories than you expended during the exercise. Many people in our study exercised an hour or day, but most did not. They were active, however.

What is exercise for one person may not be exercise for another. If you have trouble getting up and walking around the house, you will not want to be even thinking about running around the block. People have what they call the metabolic equivalent of task (MET). This is the equivalent amount of effort that someone would have to expend during an activity and is a measurement of oxygen usage. The more overweight you are, the more difficult it will be to do any given activity. If you are a healthy weight, in good physical condition, and well trained aerobically (e.g. running) and anaerobically (e.g. weight lifting or sprinting), any given exercise is going to be less difficult for you.

So, what should you do? Do the best you can, but always strive for more. If you can't walk around the block, make something toward that your goal. If you can do something that uses oxygen while you exercise, like running or biking, maybe try to go longer or faster. If you don't have any of this aerobic activity, add some. This is a common mistake among a lot of guys who lift weights. They can lift a ton, but they won't be able to catch you because they get winded. Also, if you don't do anything anaerobic, add something. Anaerobic means without air, in the same way that aerobic means with air. Weight lifting is commonly thought of as anaerobic. You don't generally do it long enough to get oxygen to your muscles. If you do a lot of repetitions (generally at a low weight) this crosses over into more aerobic activity. Weight lifting is great. It will help provide your body with strength, definition, and stronger bones. Things we all need. And don't worry, you are not going to look like a body builder without a monumental amount of effort. Those folks work super hard at it.

The other way you can provide yourself with anaerobic activity is through high intensity work-outs. This includes anything that resembles sprinting, that is, actual running, biking, or anything really fast and really hard. Sprints are great for weight loss. Like eliminating animal products, they are something that really shakes things up. They get the blood moving and activate hormones and systems that are not normally active.[135] So, if you are used to doing aerobic activity like jogging, biking, elliptical, etc., try adding something equivalent to sprints to your workout. You can do this by adding resistance or weight, or by adding speed. Sprints necessitate short bursts of energy. That is, you cannot to a true sprint for a long period of time. You want to go all out. A word of warning though: Don't do sprints unless your heart is

---

[135] Meckel Y, Eliakim A, Seraev M, Zaldivar F, Cooper DM, Sagiv M, Nemet D. The effect of a brief sprint interval exercise on growth factors and inflammatory mediators. J Strength Cond Res. 2009 Jan;23(1):225-30.

healthy, and you are used to doing aerobic activity for a while. They are hard, tiring, and are meant to make your heart work toward its max. Again, exercise is a continuum. Do the best you can but strive for more. At least, be active but strive for exercise, that is something repetitive and done for fitness. Ten minutes of brisk walking has been shown to increase your life expectancy by 1.8 years, while an hour a day of that same brisk walking can give you four and a half more years of life. If you combine both that activity level and being a normal weight, you gain a whopping 7.2 years of life on this earth than being inactive and obese.[136] The point is this: Be active to the best of your ability, be consistent, and don't eat up the progress you have made in your weight loss.

<u>Other Reasons to Make the Plunge.</u>
As if losing weight weren't reason enough to try a vegan diet, the follow is a list of other great reasons to help keep you motivated. For some people it is easier to stick with something if they feel they are doing it for someone else rather than just for themselves. See what motivates you and think of it in your times of weakness. For instance, "I want my children to have a father and not to lose their dad to heart disease the way I did," "I want the world to be a more peaceful, cleaner place," or "I don't want anything to die for me to eat, like my pet calf did on grandpa's farm." Whatever works, eating more vegetable products has many benefits for everybody.

- <u>Veganism is Great for Your Overall Health.</u>
  Vegan diets are high in nutrients. Vegetable products contain no cholesterol. They also contain fewer agricultural chemicals, and none if you eat organically.

---

[136]Steven C. Moore , Alpa V. Patel, Charles E. Matthews, Amy Berrington de Gonzalez, Yikyung Park, Hormuzd A. Katki, Martha S. Linet, Elisabete Weiderpass, Kala Visvanathan, Kathy J. Helzlsouer, Michael Thun, Susan M. Gapstur, Patricia Hartge, I-Min Lee. Leisure Time Physical Activity of Moderate to Vigorous Intensity and Mortality: A Large Pooled Cohort Analysis. PLOS Medicine. November 6, 2012.

Animal products, which are higher on the food chain, actually concentrate pesticides and herbicides which commonly are stored in fat. By eating these products, they "bioconcentrate" into your fat which your body thus stores. The same goes for many of the drugs, hormones, and chemicals given to livestock. Consumption of animals that were treated with antibiotics is an ever-increasing concern for humans in the creation of drug-resistant "superbugs." Even if you eat organic animal products (the animals themselves may have been raised organically), they still bioconcentrate whatever chemicals are already in their environment.

Vegan diets have been linked to decreased risks for cancer, heart disease, osteoporosis, kidney stones and gallstones, adult onset diabetes, multiple sclerosis, arthritis, obesity, and intestinal problems. Vegan diets are high in fiber, decreasing intestinal transit time, exposure to unwanted, undigested, or toxic material, thus cutting the risk of colorectal cancer. These fibers also help reduce the amount of cholesterol in the body and help remove it from the system.

- <u>Veganism is Great for the Environment.</u>
Environmentalist should be required to be vegans simply because vegan diets take less fuel and water to produce. It takes 78 calories of fossil fuel to produce one calorie of beef protein; 35 calories for one calorie of pork; 22 calories for one of poultry; but just one calorie of fossil fuel for one calorie of soybeans. It also takes ten times as much water to produce animal protein as it does plant protein. It takes 16 pounds of soybeans and grains to produce 1 lb. of beef and 3 to 6 lbs. to produce 1 lb. of turkey & eggs. Eating a vegan diet is thus much more efficient. In addition, the production of livestock takes a toll on our environment though the creation of excess animal

waste and destruction of the rainforests for livestock (as I am sure you have heard).

- <u>Veganism is Great for your Wallet.</u>
Not only do most vegan foods cost less than animal products, your wallet will thank you in the long run because you will have to spend less on health care and be out less on sick-time. Rely on less processed, natural foods to save the most money rather than highly processed "convenience" foods.

- <u>Veganism is Great for Your Peace of Mind.</u>
Veganism shows respect for life, love of living, and love for yourself. Religions teach: "Thou shalt not kill." They never said, "Thou shalt not kill humans; kill the rest and let God sort them out." Religion teaches mercy and forgiveness. Eastern religions teach ahimsa, nonviolence.

CHAPTER 6

MORE THINGS TO TRY ON YOUR ROAD TO WEIGHT LOSS

SUMMARY

- Try adding exercise to your program
- Eliminate obseogens.
- Don't binge. If you do, have this or any other eating disorder, ask for help and treatment.
- Veganism is the healthy, environmentally-friendly, low-cost, loving way to go.

7 INSPIRATIONAL STORIES FROM MY RESEARCH

One hundred fifty-one people responded to my study. They came from thirty-nine states, plus Canada, Saudi Arabia, Switzerland, and Australia. About half were women and about half were men.

Here is some of what they said:

I never felt better than since I became a vegan. I lost sixty-seven pounds. I never used to exercise, but now I walk or recumbent bike three or four times a week. I get most of my protein from tofu, nuts, and seeds. I drink lots of fresh vegetable juices, and carrot and celery juice with orange.

I used to eat a lot of junk food, but then I became vegetarian. I think that people who become vegetarian become much more health conscious. I try to keep my portions in check, too. I lost thirteen pounds, which was just right.

My husband and I became vegetarian at the urging of our physician due to heart disease and very high cholesterol. In eight months, he has lost twenty pounds and I have lost eighteen. We walk in the morning and bike in the evening, too. We both feel much better, though we are more wrinkled, but wrinkles are more comfortable than fat!

I had a vegan sandwich one day and thought to myself, "Those guys eat pretty well." So, I thought I would try it for thirty days. The stomach cramps I've always had disappeared. It's fifteen years later, and I wouldn't consider eating meat. I lost forty-five pounds.

I used to eat anything that wasn't nailed down. I reached over 250 pounds at my high. After that, I stopped weighing myself. So, I figure I lost at least 125 pounds. I used to eat meat and junk food, but mainly lots of dairy. Now, I am a size 8, vegan grandmother with a nice, flat tummy. I eat lots of whole grains and veggies. Learning to cook was a challenge. I have eaten fish and eggs on occasion, but the thing I found most detrimental to my health, more so than any other non-vegetarian food item, was dairy. I strictly avoid all dairy products now.

I find that eating two cups of raw fruit a day makes my skin smooth. My hair grows and inch a month! And my nails are great. I don't drink soda because I find it fattening. Processed foods in general don't burn from exercise as well as less chemical foods. Spicy foods seem to burn off, too. I lost 65 pounds. I was an overweight child, raised on a traditional diet of Twinkies, eggs, meat, processed food, and television. My parents drove me to school for fear of kidnapping. My parents couldn't understand why I was overweight and my teachers, doctors, classmates, and the school nurse were cruel. I tried lots of diets and exercise, but they didn't work. I stopped eating meat for ethical reasons and the aerobics class started to work. Even dairy products burned off better than meat, but I avoid them now, too. I heard that soft drinks and sugar lock the fat in, so I stopped that, too. I used to eat out, and you would not believe the weight I lost just by learning to eat at home. I believe that the processing and chemicals in many foods affects your metabolism. Now I walk to work and eat more organic fruits and vegetable, especially berries. The secret is vegan diet and exercise, even if you just walk.

I do yoga and am a vegan. I'm also sixty and in better health and feel better that I did twenty years ago. I became a vegetarian and then gradually a vegan. I wish I had been enlightened enough to have made this choice when much younger. I'm 21 pounds lighter.

I lost 100 pounds total and, I swear, 90 of those pounds came off in the first 90 or so days. I used to eat everything. That was 40 years ago. Now I am vegan and raw food. I eat fruits, nuts, and salad, and do yoga.

I stopped eating meat and poultry and lot fifty pounds in three years with no effort. I stopped eating fish and then became vegan and lost another twenty. I run or jog and feel great.

I used to be a lazy eater with lots of dairy and a little meat and olive oil in everything. Now I'm vegan and lost twenty pounds so far. I have lots of energy. I'm never hungry. My skin looks ten years younger and my chronic asthma has lessened considerably. You can't imagine how freeing these new eating habits are!

Since becoming vegan my cholesterol dropped as did my weight. My opinion is that conversion to unprocessed foods and elimination of meat and dairy is the easiest and most effective way to reduce personal poundage. The first person to effectively market such a program in America is going to be a millionaire!

I lost thirty pounds. Everyone noticed I was losing weight and kept telling me how nice I looked. I also used to have terrible chest pain. Now, I have none. I got away from white sugar and white flour. I eat lots of fresh fruits and vegetables, potatoes, nuts, seeds, dry beans, whole grains like brown rice, millet, oatmeal, amaranth, quinoa, and buckwheat. I quit drinking milk and eating dairy products. I just dearly love eating this way and praise the Lord for helping me find this path and ridding me of my health problems. It is a very big change to get used to. I bought a bunch of cookbooks to help. Once in a while, I have a slice of pizza with meat, but I always feel terrible afterwards. Deep fried foods also make me feel terrible. I have to get myself out of those bad habits.

I began eating a vegan diet, stopping all meat, dairy, and eggs. Now as a vegan, I weight twenty pounds less. I slipped up for a while and started eating dairy and eggs again, and my weight went up eight pounds. Now I've started a vegan diet again and the weight is coming off at a rate of about a pound every four days. I've also cut out most white sugar recently. As an interesting side note, I used to get headaches. Cutting out the dairy and eggs has decreased them significantly. They decreased even more when I cut out the sugar. Thanks! Hope this helps.

I don't really worry about what I eat now. I just eat vegan foods my body is craving. I never get sick and I'm stronger and more alert and less tired than I used to be when I was a flesh eater.

So far, I have lost 23 pounds. I haven't been doing any real exercise program since I have two small children. I shop carefully and we do not use any boxed cereals. I've really gotten into making my own homemade bread.

I've lost 35 pounds so far. I am seven or eight pounds from my ideal weight. I have lost weight before. This has been so easy. I eat what I want (that is vegan) and the weight falls off. I hope this information helps someone else who has fought with weight loss.

I will gladly share my continuing success story. I started vegetarianism for health reasons. My cholesterol was 260 and dieting didn't work. I was also hypertensive and overweight. I read an article about a woman who was overweight but achieved a healthy weight and good health on a vegetarian diet. I decided that my husband and I would give it a try. I couldn't control my intake of meat, chicken, and fish, so I decided to eliminate all three thereby avoiding any temptation to binge on these high cholesterol foods. I started finding recipes and cutting down on dairy and eggs.

My cholesterol has come down and I have lost 66 pounds in a little over a year. My doctor is pleased with my progress. I am eating vegetable, grains, beans, rice, pasta, fruit, and veggie burgers. I still have been trying to limit my food intake and keep a food diary since I still think I gain weight rapidly.

What an interesting project! Yes, definitely I believe that a veg. diet in a fantastic way to lose/control weight. I gave up my morning coffee and donuts. I loved them but I can't imagine ingesting such a disgusting thing now —white flour, sugar, and rancid oil. I also loved chocolate, pie, and ice cream, but now these things are unbearably sweet. I gave up sausage and bacon and deep-fried stuff. No more potato chips and soda. I love food — good whole, natural veg food. I don't eat a lot of fat, so I can eat a lot. Everyone is always amazed how much I can eat, and they never cease expressing their profound dismay at how "slender" I am. I am very lucky to have discovered how to control my weight. Up until the time I stopped eating meat, I always had to "fight" to maintain my weight. Now I'm always full and satisfied, and not fat! Good luck with your project.

I lost 14 pounds over a three-month period when I stopped eating dairy products. I previously had given up meat without much effect. The weight loss was not intentional, but it was welcome. I've stayed that weight ever since. I got rid of the extra pounds I put on when I stopped smoking.

Alcohol, cigarettes, pills, and food were my devils. I blew up to 280 pounds and was miserable. I got so sick that I almost died. I woke up one morning and found Jesus Christ and a new life. I knew I had been dying little by little. I threw out all of the alcohol, the cigarettes, the pills, and all the junk I was eating and vowed to whip the devil's (bleep). I ripped out all the demons by the roots — all on the first day. It was thirty days of hell. I drank water, ate fruits and vegetables, and walked — all day long. In 130 days, I lost 125 pounds. I lost almost a pound a day except for the last five days. It took longer to lose that last 2 ½ pounds. I learned how to cook and how to get all of the necessary nutrients on a pure vegetarian diet. Now I am a dynamic cook. Today, over five years later I feel like a zillion dollars. Had I not cleaned out my blood and purified it with "healing foods" I would never had the brains to be what I am today. God bless you, sister. If you know anybody with booze, pills, smokes, meat, etc., please share this with them and I will convert them to the "Fountain of Youth." I have drive, and food and fresh air. All I can say is a vegetarian vegan is a winner all the way. I put away Lucifer right on his butt. Read the King

James Bible, Genesis 1:29 and 1:30. You'll see where the Seventh Day Adventists got their vegetarian medical minds from!

"And God said, Behold, I have given you every herb bearing seed, which is upon the face of all the earth, and every tree, in which is the fruit of a tree yielding seed; to you it shall be for meat." King James Bible, Genesis 1:29

"And to every beast of the earth, and to every fowl of the air, and to everything that creepeth upon the earth, wherein there is life, I have given every green herb for meat: and it was so." King James Bible, Genesis 1:30

"Whoever slaughters an ox is like one who slays a man; whoever sacrifices a lamb is like one who breaks a dog's neck;..." Isaiah 66:3

I have lost 75 pounds in the last year and a half. There was a gradual loss of weight, and the rate picked up as I moved more toward veganism. Initially, I still ate fish. Then I stopped, but I was still eating copious amounts of dairy products, so I cut back on that, too. Now, it is rare for me to eat any eggs or dairy. I was one of those "French fry" vegetarians for a while. Now, I'm cutting out that extra fat, too.

At first, I ate everything with my family except the meat. Then I started bringing home cookbooks from the library. My weight has dropped 20 pounds thus far and my cholesterol has dropped 50 points. I am convinced that the menstrual problems I was having were from the hormones in the meat, since they have almost entirely cleared up. I do feel better, not as sluggish, and I'm excited about the new changes in my diet.

So far, I have lost 80 pounds since becoming a vegetarian, but I was still really eating a high fat diet. Now I have started cutting out the eggs and am taking very little milk, and the weight seems to be coming off faster.

So far, I have lost 16 pounds, but I really have a long way to go yet. Then again, it has only been two months. I have been eating beans, rice, whole wheat bread, vegetables, and fruits. I usually have oatmeal for breakfast, a vegetable sandwich for lunch, and pasta and beans for dinner. So far so good. Wish me strength for the long haul!

I became an ovo-lactovegetarian for ethical reasons and my decision was not looked upon with pleasure by my parents. I was doing it for ethical/spiritual reasons, but I wanted to be a healthy vegetarian. I read a lot! I really only ate eggs and dairy when we were out to eat. Then I stopped eating eggs and dairy altogether becoming a vegan. No compromise. I was always overweight, so years ago I learned to accept my weight, as well as myself, and my weight actually did not bother me at all. I was a size 28. When I became a vegetarian I didn't even enter my mind that I might lose weight. However, several weeks into my "change," I realized that not only did I feel great, my sinus problems disappeared, and my clothes felt looser. I got on the scale and found out how much I weighed. I really didn't know. I had stopped weighing myself years ago. From then on, I monitored my weight loss. The pounds literally fell off. Gradually, I began exercising, walking daily and lifting a few free weights at home, cheap exercise. It took me 16 months to plateau 155 pounds later! That was 1 ½ years ago. I seldom weight myself now, but it changes by no more than one or two pounds up and down. I have no problem maintaining my weight. I am pretty used to it now. What seems most odd in to have people tell me I'm skinny. They freak out when they learn I lost 155 pounds! I went from a size 28 to a size 6, and my bra was a 48DD. Now it is a 34A! I don't miss that at all!

I came from a heavy meat-eating family where every meal was centered around meat. I became vegan seven months ago with my fiancé for environmental reasons. At first, we didn't know just what to eat, but now we are having all kinds of new recipes. In a few short months, I lost 18 pounds and my fiancée lost 15! We feel great and have a lot of energy. My hair doesn't break, and my nails don't chip. My skin is radiant and now I have regular menstrual cycles. I wouldn't go back to the fatty, unhealthy lifestyle of meat eating for anything.

I went to a health institute to lose weight on a pure vegetarian diet and lost 20 pounds in a short period of time. At home, I lost 12 more, for a total of 32 pounds. I feel much better, have lots of energy, and no food cravings nor heart burn. I am eating fruit, vegetables, beans, sprouts, grains, and seeds, all vegan. So far, so good.

I have lost 24 ½ pounds in 4 ½ months since becoming vegan. I became vegetarian in college but like a college student with bagels smothered in cream cheese, cheddar cheese and avocado sandwiches, huge Mexican bean and cheese burritos with sour cream, ice cream, and, of course, beer. When I became vegetarian, I actually gained ten pounds because I ate so mush, especially dairy. Now I have become vegan and that extra weight has come off. I am thrilled to have lost the weight. I look and feel better. Everyone in my family is so proud of me.

I have lost 14 pounds since becoming mostly vegan. I still have a little egg white and less than a cup of nonfat milk daily. I decided to change my eating habits for health reasons, not to lose weight. The weight loss has been an excellent and unexpected bonus to my new-found self.

When I read that you were looking for people who had lost weight on a vegetarian diet, I had to write. I am very happy that someone besides myself has taken an interest in the weight loss benefits from a vegetarian diet.

I lost weight when I became a vegetarian because of a boyfriend. I hated eggs and was allergic to dairy, so I really was a vegan. I went from 170 pounds to 136 pounds. After we broke-up, I became a meat eater again just to spite him, but I also went back up to 170 pounds. Later, I decided to become vegetarian again on my own and quickly lost the weight. I should have realized I should have been a vegetarian all along. I say that weight is hereditary which one cannot totally control. I wish doctors could realize that my family is either vegetarian or obese. My grandmother was vegetarian, and the rest of the family was either vegetarian or obese. They thought I would die from being vegan since I didn't eat eggs and was allergic to dairy. Later, I found a dietitian that said I would be fine. I never liked meat that much and don't miss it. My blood pressure used to be high, but now it is normal. I do aerobic and avoid coffee and alcohol. I used to also have fatty skin cysts which went away. I will never eat meat again.

I do not consider my new eating habits a "diet." I eat as much as I want. The difference is what I eat, and the results have been spectacular. I lost 100 pounds and went from a size 22 jeans to a size 10. I would never make the simplistic claim that a vegetarian regimen is a cure-all, but it played a key role in the new slimmer reflection I see in the mirror.

So far, I have lost 50 pounds on a vegan diet. I have been on it for the last six months and I plan to stay on it since I have another 50 pounds to lose. I have been averaging 6 to 8 pounds loss after an initial 20 pounds in in the first 6 weeks. I am eating cereal, beans, brown rice, salsa, corn tortillas, corn, fresh fruits and vegetables, and low-fat soy milk on my cereal. I'm avoiding caffeine and am exercising at least three times a week.

I have changed my diet slowly over the past five years. First, I cut down on red meat, then chicken and fish. I spent about a year eating meat or fish only once per week. Then, I cut them out completely. I drastically cut down on my consumption of cheese, other dairy, and eggs. Now, I eat them very infrequently. Losing weight was never my goal, but I lost 20 pounds and it has remained there for the past year with no other change in my lifestyle. Losing weight was a welcome side effect.

I lost 23 pounds after cutting out all red meat, chicken, fish, every meat. My energy level is up, my metabolism is at an all-time high, and my body fat continues to drop!

I used to weigh 112 pounds when I was young but put on weight as I got older and got up to 132 pounds. I would go on a diet and lose some weight now and again, but never got down to my youthful weight. Seven years ago, I became aware of the suffering I was indirectly inflicting on animal by continuing to eat them. For that reason, I became vegetarian. Slowly, my weight dropped until I reached my old 112 pounds and my weight never went lower. Once I reached the 112, the weight loss stopped even though at one point I had been concerned that if I continued to lose a few pounds every year I would be too thin, but that has not happened.

My mother, grandmother, and I all cut out the meat. I lost 30 pounds, my mother lost 40 pounds, and my grandmother has lost 100 pounds. We barely eat meat at all anymore. I use seitan and veggie burgers, and don't use any dairy products.

I have lost 20 pounds in nine months since becoming vegetarian. I cut out the colas and alcohol as well. Following my decision to stop eating meat, I noticed a profound difference in the way my clothing fit and how I looked in the mirror.

After 20 years of trying to lose weight, I am so thrilled and grateful about losing weight since becoming a vegetarian. I can hardly call it a diet in the usual meaning of the word. I am never stuffed, but still satisfied. I love to cook and make my recipes vegan. I had gained weight from medication and no diet of any kind helped. I stopped eating meat gradually, using only seafood and poultry, and then gradually eliminated those as well. After being on vacation in South East Asia, I realized that I was eating as a vegan, and had lost weight. I hadn't gotten sick, the way everyone else on the trip had either. So far in the past seven months, I have lost 17 pounds. Needless to add, I am, indeed, a happy person. Most of the restaurants in our area cater to vegan, too. If people would take a gradual approach to being a vegetarian then vegan, as I did, it is not at all difficult.

I have been a vegetarian for over 20 years but never really noticed a big difference in my weight. Now that I have crossed over completely — What a difference! I wasn't trying to lose weight becoming a vegan, but it is a nice bonus. I feel great!

In five months, I have lost 30 pounds and my cholesterol is going down. I am enjoying reading about all of the health benefits and trying recipes. Still going strong, I've got a ways to go.

In the past year I have lost ten pounds with no extra effort. All I did was become a vegan.

Ten years ago, I had three blocked arteries and cardiac catheterization. My doctor made me change everything. I quit smoking, started doing yoga for exercise every day, and became a strict vegetarian. My cholesterol was 299 and quickly dropped to 153 without the use of medication. I lost 32 pounds without even trying. I eat all the time, but I eat the right foods. I really felt that I had to continue this program for the rest of my life. I feel like a 20-year-old now. I feel wonderful. I know that becoming a vegan prevented me from having to have a bi-pass.

I started a vegan diet with a friend. We said we would switch for 30 days for health reasons. I wasn't really sick, but I didn't have much energy and generally wanted to regain control over my life. I felt so good after the month that I stayed on the diet. It has been a year now and I have lost 50 pounds. I feel better than ever before physically. This in turn has brought about very positive changes emotionally and spiritually as well. Losing weight was never my main objective, but obviously I needed to do so.

I've lost 30 pounds in the last year with very little effort since becoming vegetarian. I still have maybe 25 to go. The biggest change for me came when I stopped eating fast food. I also really started reading labels. I have no desire to eat meat now. In fact, the longer I'm vegetarian, the more meat disgusts me.

Becoming vegetarian made me cut down on fats and sugars. I lost 32 pounds. I've found that I do best when I only eat at meal times and I'm walking daily.

I dropped 37 pounds in four months when I became a strict vegetarian. I went from having a pot belly to slim. I gradually stopped eating red meat, then chicken and fish, and most of the eggs and milk. I also stopped drinking too much beer. I ate lots of fiber and started exercising — walking and weight lifting a few times a week. I could not have done this without becoming a vegetarian. In fairness, I did a lot of other things, too, but the vegetarian diet was the cornerstone. I have come to see this whole topic as a three-legged stool — diet, physical conditioning, and emotional and mental health. You absolutely have to work on all three, but diet is more than half of it. After the diet, the rest comes much easier.

I became vegetarian for moral reasons. This made it very easy to stick to the diet. Over the course of three years I have lost 25 pounds and now am very interested in the health benefits of becoming vegetarian.

In the last 20 days, I have lost 18 pounds. I used to eat burgers, pizza, and tacos most days of the week. After reading an animal rights book about where beef comes from, I felt so bad. Sad. I decided to become vegetarian. The first few days, I had a headache and body pains. The second week, I craved sweets. Now, I feel good and am having far fewer cravings. I plan on sticking with it. I have about 60 more pounds to go, and I feel it is really doable. Having the motivation that I am helping animals at the same time I am becoming healthier really helps.

Since I have cut meat out of my diet, I have lot 20 pounds in 6 months. I know cutting meat from my diet has kept me slim and more aware of my body weight.

I have lost 45 pounds since becoming a vegetarian. For exercise, I do walking or hatha yoga most days of the week.

I've lost 10 pounds since becoming a vegetarian – the rest of me is muscle.

I've lost 13 pounds since becoming a vegetarian. My exercise program is light – walking, tai chi, and sometimes weights.

I lost 10 pounds when I became a vegetarian. My right kidney had bothered me. After becoming a vegetarian a while, my hay fever and kidney problems were gone. I don't get sick. During an examination at the Veterans' Hospital one of two of the physicians told me, "You are in better shape than we are." I was 85. Now I am 92 – Still no problems. I never thought I had much of a weight problem. I just didn't want to get sick. Vegetarianism is a preventative lifestyle!

I became a pure vegetarian because I believed it was wrong to eat animal products. I initially lost 10 pounds, but after my initial weight loss, my weight has stayed the same for 25 years. I am 82 now.

I lost 90 pounds when I became a vegetarian. My weight has crept up though over the years. I am not watching things as closely as I am getting older, and I sometimes eat whatever I can get a hand on, including chicken. I'm still 30 pounds lighter than my heaviest weight though, and life has been very stressful.

I lost 35 pounds when I became a vegetarian.

I lost 42 pounds when I became a vegetarian. My activity level was high then, and it still is now, so the weight loss can all be attributed to the diet.

I became a vegan entirely last winter. No meat, dairy. No sugar or alcohol. I have lost 50 pounds in eight months. I don't think I will have a problem keeping the weight off either.

I stopped eating meat, fish, eggs, milk products, and added oils two months ago. So far, I have lost 16 pounds. I chose this eating program for a general health improvement, not primarily for weight loss, but the weight loss is also an obvious health benefit. I do yoga and vegetarianism is one of their major tenants, so I wanted to practice yoga fully.

After we got married, our weights shot up. Making meats was easy and so was going out to eat. Eventually, we both tried a popular magazine's low-calorie diet. "I am always hungry," my husband complained. I was hungry, too. We tried Atkins. He called it "carbohydrate intolerance." We had one-inch steaks slathered with butter, greasy chicken, and pork chops sizzling in their own lard. I lost 10 pounds and my husband lost 25. But our digestive systems were not functioning properly. We couldn't keep it up, so that diet ended, and we regained the weight we had lost. I started reading about the environmental concerns of meat production and began to think that animal products were unnecessary. How could we feed our cows the grains that could feed the starving world? I started to think that animal products might be unhealthy, too. My husband and I both became pure vegetarians. It has been ten years now and not only did we lose that extra weight, but we have kept it off the whole ten years without a struggle. We don't find the diet limiting. It has opened us to new ideas, foods, and recipes.

I was one of those few ovo-lacto-vegetarians who were way too fat. I obviously ate too much, especially dairy products. Three months ago, I decided to become vegan. Since then, I have lost 17 pounds. In addition to changing my diet, I started walking for a total of 2 ½ hours a week and lift weights twice a week. My body has definitely firmed-up. I feel great, have a lot of stamina, and am not hungry.

When I became vegan, I lost 20 pounds. The last time I had ice cream, my ankles got swollen (so I won't do that again). I feel that dairy products and sugar are terrible for me. I don't get sick, which I like very much.

I lost 10 pounds by slowly cutting out red meat, poultry, and fish over the last year.

I tried Weight Watchers and after 6 months of hard work, I only lost 3 pounds. I then went to a naturopath who put me on a vegetarian diet. I've lost 20 pounds. I don't eat dairy. I gain weight when I start eating them.

I have lost 17 pounds since becoming a vegetarian. I have been eating dairy products but have been avoiding eggs. I have lost 1 to 1 ½ pounds a week so far, which is good since I have been trying to lose 30 pounds for the last 30 years. What I discovered that changed my way of eating was how much even a small amount (or what I considered a small amount) of fat could undo and otherwise good diet. I am a little bit hungry, but not too bad. I plan to stick with it.

I've definitely lost weight since becoming a vegetarian, and it has stayed off for the past year.

My wife and I lost weight when we became vegetarians for ethical concerns. We have found though that telling others about the ethical and environmental concerns that made us switch is a good way to lose friends. They listen though when we talk about health concerns.

I stopped eating meat, fish, chicken, and desserts six months ago. I started eating desserts again after three months. I am eating some dairy and an egg or two a week. I have lost 10 pounds.

I lost 5 pounds when I became vegetarian. I lost 3 more when I became vegan. Now I'm a good weight.

I was too heavy to start with but when I stopped smoking, I gained 34 pounds. I decided to become vegetarian and then vegan. In the past eight months I have lost 32 pounds. I do fall off the wagon periodically, but when I do, I feel slightly nauseous (especially from a fatty meal) and the food really isn't as tasty as my mind seems to remember. I recommend the vegetarian/vegan diet as a gradual, steady way to lose weight.

I have lost 40 pounds since becoming vegan. I find that I have a good energy level and feel good. I have a regular hatha yoga and meditation practice. I walk and sometimes swim. I am eating salads, seeds, grains, veggies, and lots of fruit. I like having a lot of raw food. There is no doubt in my mind that a vegetarian diet with much raw food, regular yoga, lots of sunshine, and outdoor activity has greatly enhanced my health and well-being.

I've lost 20 pounds by becoming vegan. It has stayed off for the past year and only ever goes up or down a pound or two. I am 98 percent vegan. I only ever eat some eggs or dairy when it is in a baked good that I did not make myself.

I have lost 9 pounds in the past two months by eliminating meats and significantly lowering my intake of eggs and dairy.

When I was 13 years old, I had a significant weight problem. I had hypoglycemia and very high cholesterol. My doctor made me go on a no meat, no dairy, no sugar diet. I hated it at the time, but I was terrified by the doctor's speech on good nutrition, so I followed it religiously. Now, over ten years later, I am healthy and slim. I have a little dairy or sugar on occasion, but I will forever be a vegetarian. I feel great!

We became vegan and also cut out added oils, salt, caffeine, soda, refined sugar, and white flour. My husband was always very active and has always run for an hour a day but could never lose weight. Now he has lost 31 pounds and I have lost 8. So many people ask us how we did it and we don't feel like we are depriving ourselves of all the things we used to love. Once you get used to this way of eating, your tastes actually change because you feel so good about the foods you are putting in your body, you don't ever crave the "other" stuff. At least that is what we found to be true.

I gave up meat and eggs for Krishna. I lost 10 pounds in the last month since my conversion. I have also cut way down on fat and sugar.

I wanted to be a vegetarian when I was younger, but my parents would not let me until I was out on my own. As I got older, I had horrible stomach aches and fatigue. I decided to become a total vegetarian when a friend thought this would help. (I hesitate to use the word vegan since I do use leather.) I have also gotten rid of refined sugar and white flour. Since then, I definitely feel more energetic and my moods are much better. Without even trying, I lost 10 pounds, which was perfect. I've always walked daily, so that did not change. What was so surprising was that the area that I lost the most was my thighs.

In the last two months, I have lost an unbelievable 22 pounds from giving up meat, fish, poultry, and shellfish!

When I became a vegetarian, I lost 25 pounds in 3 months. It has stayed off for the past 5 years. I cut out all animal flesh and the chips, cookies, and chocolate I was eating. I eat vegetables, grains, cereals, breads, and tons of fruit which I love.

In the last two months, my husband lost 30 pounds and I lost 10 by becoming vegetarian. We both feel great!

I lost 30 pounds over an 18-month period when I gradually eliminated all animal products from my diet. I hope that people will come to realize that starvation diets and pills are not the way to go for long-lasting weight loss.

I was a very unhealthy vegetarian at 200 pounds. I didn't believe that people should eat meat for their own satisfaction. Cheese pizza, French fries, and fatty foods were the only things in my diet. Now I have educated myself about health and have lost 88 pounds on a healthy, low fat, vegan diet.

You don't know what it feels like to be sick for 33 years. My waist was fat. My neck was fat. It took all the energy I could muster to get out of bed and go to work. My energy was zero. One day I discovered a raw food, vegan diet and a week later I felt a sudden drastic change. I never felt this before in my life and it was in my body and my mind. I lost 90 pounds! My skin tightened. I never had any loose skin. I never counted any calories and I still love to eat. I also had enough energy that I started walking to work. I was a new person. That was 33 years ago.

Not only have I become a vegetarian, but I have severely reduced the amount of fat and sugar that I eat. So far, I have lost 20 pounds.

I've lost 40 pounds becoming predominantly a raw food vegan a year ago. My cholesterol is now in the healthy range.

In the past 5 months, I have lost 20 pounds by becoming an almost-vegan. The weight is staying off!

When I first became a vegetarian, I lost 10 pounds, but I was relying on cheese too much for protein that I was supposedly lacking. Then I completely cut out eggs and dairy and have lost the last 15 pounds almost effortlessly.

I had multiple problems with pregnancies and arthritis in my fingers and hips. First, I decided to give up dairy, then meat and other animal products. Now, I have lost 118 pounds. People comment on how clear my skin and eyes look. The arthritis is gone. It has been 2 years, and I am hopeful for other things now, too.

My professor had us do a three-day food diary and analyze it on the computer. She was amazed how balanced and complete my vegan diet was.

I lost five pounds a month after becoming a vegetarian. Then I cut out all the dairy products. In total, I lost 25 pounds and I have maintained my weight effortlessly since then. I love ethnic food and I hate to say it, but I still eat candy.

I became a vegetarian when I found out I was sick. So far, I have lost 110 pounds. I still have more to go. The diet is totally manageable. I have found that weight loss has little to do with what you don't eat, but rather with how you educate yourself and change your habits concerning what you do eat. I hope that your research will provide people with more information to make healthy choices.

I have had so many children and my weight has fluctuated up and down so much. This last time a nurse suggested that I become vegetarian to help control my weight and make my homebirth easier.

I gave up drugs of all kinds, cigarettes, and alcohol, and became a vegetarian 5 years ago. When I first started looking for the truth in nutrition, I changed my diet. I have a higher degree of energy than ever before and love running now. I have lost 44 pounds and it has stayed off that 5 years.

I changed my diet after reading about PMS and have lost 10 pounds on a vegetarian diet.

When I became a vegetarian, I ate a lot of eggs and milk. My weight stayed the same. Eight months ago, I cut out all of the dairy. The weight just fell off me. I lost 28 pounds. My husband lost weight, too, but he has a hard time not straying. I think that the big killer is milk.

I was upset at the continued destruction of the environment for meat production, especially the destruction of the rain forest for cheap beef. When I became vegetarian, I gradually lost 30 pounds over the course of time I adopted the diet with my wife. Living overseas, we were used to shopping daily and eating many fruits and vegetables. We have really come to love both Indian and Pakistani food.

I lost 45 pounds when I stopped all meat. That was 3 years ago.

I have lost 110 pounds since becoming a vegetarian. I eat a lot of fruit and vegetables. I do not drink milk nor take any sugar.

I've lost 80 pounds in 7 months since becoming a dairy-free vegetarian. I still plan on getting rid of another 60.

Four years ago, my cholesterol was 330 and my doctor said to stop eating red meat. Little by little, I cut back until soon I did not like it. In quick succession, poultry and fish became distasteful, and I became an unwitting vegetarian. I hardly ever have a little milk or cheese. My cholesterol is now 180, I went through menopause with no problem, and I am 80 pounds lighter.

I changed my diet radically after having an emergency triple bypass. I thought I was healthy, since I am only 55, but apparently my body thought differently. I have become vegetarian and lost 16 pounds thus far.

All of my life I was overweight and ate a heavy breakfast. My diet included milk, meat, eggs, and late dinners. I gradually started becoming vegetarian and quickly lost 40 pounds. This motivated me to be more particular about what I ate eliminating all meat, dairy, and eggs. Now I have lost 70 pounds. I try to never limit the amount I eat so I don't get hungry. I like to eat. I am thrilled that I don't have to worry about my weight. It seems to me we just need to eat food as God gave it to us.

I became a vegetarian to become healthier, not necessarily to lose weight. The biggest change though has been giving up dairy products. I have lost 20 pounds. I have never felt better or had more energy in my life.

I never liked meat and needed to lose weight so 5 months ago I started a vegetarian diet. I don't eat eggs but do have some non-fat dairy. I have lost 33 pounds in such a short period of time. Of course, I don't fry anything. I love whole wheat bagels, fruit, vegetables, brown rice, and black beans. I am so excited about my new way of eating. I love it!

My husband used to live on fast food and donuts. Now he is vegetarian and has lost 30 pounds in 3 months.

I've lost 10 pounds by becoming vegetarian. I still eat dairy and eggs in cookies and pies though.

In school I did a research paper on meat and the slaughtering of animals. I thus decided to become a vegetarian. I have lost 30 pounds. My final decision to stay vegetarian was for health reasons. I have become very concerned about what I put in my body. After all, you are what you eat!

I was a "pseudo-vegetarian" for many years eating everything but beef and pork. My weight continued to go up. When I turned 50 my weight was over 200 and my cholesterol was 349. Since then my husband and I have eliminated all animal products. I use soy and rice milk for cooking. I've been canning my own vegetables and doing freezing too in an attempt to limit as many food additives as possible. I've been feeling so good I started exercising most days of the week – which I never did before. In the last 6 months, I have lost 36 pounds, my blood pressure has dropped 20 points, and I don't know about my cholesterol yet. I have made no effort to count calories or grams fat or cholesterol. I do not intentionally restrict my intake of desserts. I feel more energized and have become a creative and inspired cook. I actually delight in the artistry of color and texture experienced in my diet. My husband has lost 30 pounds. We have expectations of losing another 20 or 30.

Since stopping eating all animal products I have lost 28 pounds in the last 5 months with the majority of weight coming off in the first 3 months.

When I grew up, we had meat of every sort from hunting. My diet consisted of meat, bacon, and sausage at every meal, plus biscuits and gravy, dumplings, and canned vegetables. When I got married, it was the same, only much of the food was fried. Now that the kids are grown, and I am vegetarian, there is no greasy layer on everything in my kitchen and it smells clean. Even when it is messy, I only have to take the trash out once a week. It doesn't smell ever. The best thing is that I am slim and healthier than ever. When you have your health, you have everything.

Since I became vegan, I have lost 27 pounds and my wife has lost 19.

I am a newly slim vegan, but I feel I am on my way. I lost 37 pounds so far and still have more to go.

I was an ovo-lactovegetarian for over 12 years but became a vegan 7 months ago. I also gave up white sugar because I heard it is filtered through charred animal bones for purification. Since then I have lost 27 pounds. I've been overweight almost all of my adult life. Although I've always tried to eat a low-fat diet, I've never had the kind of results that I've had since becoming a vegan. My diet is now naturally low-fat, and I don't have to "make allowances" for cheese, eggs, etc. This is probably why I had more trouble losing weight as an ovo-lactovegetarian. I thought I could compensate for all that cheese.

No diet or exercise program worked for me until I became a vegetarian. I have lost 40 pounds. I didn't put any effort into trying to lose weight. All I did was concentrate on maintaining a meatless diet. The weight has dropped off with no struggle to keep it off. Now I am at my best. I look good and feel good. I have more energy than ever before. I have always had a weak back, but without that extra weight, I no longer have backaches.

I stopped eating all animal products one month ago and have lost 12 pounds.

I stopped all animal products to try to get rid of ovarian cysts that are extremely painful. So far, so good. I feel better, more energy, and have lost 12 pounds.

My friend told me that when he was on a vegan diet, his blood pressure went from 190/110 to 120/80 and his cholesterol went from 250 to 150. At first, I disregarded it. I was a burger person. Years later, I decided to give it a try. I had used fruits and vegetables to lose weight before, so I thought I would give veganism a try. My blood pressure went from 180/100 to 120/80 and my cholesterol went from 180 to 130. I've lost 55 pounds.

Although my weight loss has been minimal (10 pounds) on a vegetarian diet, the health effects have been vast.

My mother had a triple bi-pass in her early forties and my aunt died of a stroke also in her early forties. Now in my mid-forties, my doctor told me I was facing the same possibility based on my bloodwork. I didn't want to wind up like the other women in my family, so I became vegan. Two months later, I had my blood drawn again. This time the bloodwork says, "Excellent, continue with diet." I've lost 13 pounds. Now I knew being a vegan was going to be a life-time commitment. The doctor said he is going to reduce my medication when I lose a little more weight. I feel like a real winner, full of energy and vitality.

It has been a year since losing 30 pounds on a vegan diet. My cholesterol has gone from 230 to 160. The weight seemingly fell off my body. I don't feel the need to sleep so much now either.

I lost 35 pounds in 8 months by eliminating all animal products and alcohol. I have not tried to limit the volume of food I have consumed.

My husband and I got sick one night from food poisoning from beef tacos, and that was it. I could not eat it anymore. I stopped eating beef, chicken, and eggs. My weakness are ice cream and cheese, but I only eat them once in a great while. In 9 months, I have lost 45 pounds. I have never looked or felt better. Best of all, it really wasn't an effort for me because the idea of animal products in general became disgusting to me.

I stopped eating seafood and pork since I didn't eat much of them anyway. Next came chicken and red meat, then dairy and eggs. I've been a full vegan for 5 months and have lost 30 pounds. In fact, I had lost a little bit more, but then decided I should probably eat bigger portions since I am a muscular guy.

CHAPTER 7

INSPIRATIONAL STORIES FROM MY RESEARCH

SUMMARY

- Find a friend in these stories to use as inspiration.
- Stick with it; it works.
- Find a buddy for support amongst your friends and family, or maybe start your own weight loss group.

8 HOW TO RUN A WEIGHT LOSS GROUP

One of the best things that anyone can do on their journey is have a support group. From my previous, original research into resilience in breastfeeding mothers, the women that overcame hardships were more likely to have a plan and a group of people to help. It doesn't matter what kind of obstacle you have. If you have a plan and a support group, just about anything can be overcome. Weight loss is no different: With a plan and support, things can happen.

The one thing that is different though is that hopefully by now, from reading this book, reading about how others have used a vegan diet successfully for achieving a healthy weight, and trying some of the ideas in this book, you have seen some proof of the efficacy of veganism for health and well-being. Because of this you may be so inspired to help others and spread the good news. One of the best ways you can do this is by starting a vegan weight loss support group.

You don't have to be a nutritionist to do this. You are holding all the tools you need right here in your hands.

First, come up with a place where you might meet and get some friends together to join you. You might meet in your house or at a friend's place. You could try your church or other space that might have a meeting room available. You might try a local library, a café, or a health-minded doctor's office (like my husband's chiropractic office) or hospital community room. I suggest not getting together around food. Sometimes it seems that everything we do that is social revolves around food and eating. Make this something that doesn't or maybe just have out drinks. Having food also makes it a little too difficult sometimes for the organizers. Make it easy on everyone, including yourself, so everybody, including you, will keep coming.

After you have a place and a couple core people that you know will come, have all of you try to round up a few more folks. A support group is for just that, support. Don't try to go it alone. You need support and encouragement, too. Make sure you have at least one buddy that will be there to help be "in charge." Try spreading the news within your social media networks. There are also many free places to advertise online for free community events like Craig's List and your local television stations or newspapers.

Think about your agenda for your meeting. I like to go by a certain format that builds relationships, is educational, and has a motivational effect. I suggest dividing your meeting into the following time segments:

1. Gathering

    A few things are very helpful to have at every meeting include name tags, little notebooks or paper, pens or pencils, an electronic scale that will weigh larger masses (not all scales will accommodate larger individuals so you want to try to provide attendees with a scale where they can at least weight themselves periodically at your meetings).

    While you are waiting for everyone to come, greet people as they enter. Be the consummate host. I believe this means helping everyone get a name tag and I like to give everyone a little, pocket-sized notebook or paper and a pen so that they can take notes later if they want. Greet everyone coming in. Tell them your name and who you are. Try to remember their name and make yourself a little cheat-sheet somewhere to help; something like, "Suzie is a short curly blonde; Dave has glasses and a big beard." Get people to put on name tags, too. Also, try your best to find out something about them. This is for general interest and socializing, but also so that you can help facilitate introductions. Don't let anyone stand alone isolated. They won't come back. Think about what people have in common or something interesting about them and introduce them to others to help them get the ball rolling in conversation, even if you have to leave to help somewhere else. The point is you want people to build friendships; you want them to build community.

When you feel that everyone that is going to show is there, introduce yourself again to the group and ask everyone to take a seat to start the next phase of your meeting.

2. Group Introductions

You needn't do this every single meeting, but you should at least do a quick round of names each time. Group leaders tend to get sloppy about this sometimes. Just because you know everyone's names, it doesn't mean everyone else does. Maybe they came a few times, but now they are getting back into it. Don't expect people to remember. Again, make it easy on people and get in a habit of wearing name tags and making introductions.

For your first meeting, however, it is especially important to have everyone introduce themselves. Start with yourself and a general welcome and then go around the room with introductions. Say who you are, what you hope to gain or learn from coming to the group, and maybe something about your life especially as it relates to your health and weight. Give everyone time. We all can learn from each other. When you make your way around back to you as the group leader, introduce yourself again this time with a little more details and then tell them about the structure of the meetings and what to expect. I suggest following with the three components: 1) information and learning, 2) visualizing, and (3) questions, sharing, and follow-up.

3. Information and Learning

For this section you will want to focus on a particular topic concerning diet and health. When you do your advertising, you will want to let people know the topic for the evening. Some folks may not be interested in recipes, but they might be interested in weight's relation to cancer for instance. Mix-up your topics so it keeps things interesting. Now, this is where this book comes in. Pick a section of this book to go over. Pick a few pages to either read or give you a general outline about what to talk about. For example, maybe you want to talk about the section "Serious Symptoms to Address Before You Start." You can either read this section verbatim or use it as your notes to talk off the top of your head. This will of course depend on how familiar you are with the subject. One way of teaching that tends to be very motivational is giving people the bad things to think about (the consequences) and then giving them the things that they can do to avoid these problems. These are your suggested action plans. Here you will want to talk about some aspect of "going vegan" that can help. Maybe you want to talk about how and why to cut back on everything "white" (flour, milk, sugar, etc.). Again pick a section in the book to read and go over. Feel free to mark up your book and write down what you want to say. It's your after all and it will make you a much stronger more competent group leader.

At the end of this section of the meeting have everyone write down at least one thing that they are willing to do to move towards their health goals. Even little steps add up. Encourage everyone to pick a little something they learned or thought of while listening, then go onto visualizing.

4. Visualizing

Visualizing is a very important step in helping people achieve their goals. If you have picked a topic from "Reclaiming Yourself Physically & Mentally," feel free to read directly. You could also just speak from the heart or ask participants to simply visualize (preferably with their eyes closed) what they don't want to happen, then replace it by erasing the mental image they had with a new, better outcome as a result of the positive action plan and steps that they have told themselves they will take. The idea is that you want to give some time with guided imagery and then let the individual have time to reflect and have time to think.

5. Question, Sharing, and Follow-up

Take this time for sharing. There might be some questions. If you can answer them fine. If not, maybe someone else in the group can or you will get back to them at the next meeting with an answer. Have people do some sharing about what they thought, felt, and what they thought they could change. You don't have to be in charge all the time. Let the conversation go where it might. If people get off the subject, it is your job as the group leader to bring them back to the topic at hand. Tell folks about the next meeting and that there is a scale available for use, then let the group open to socializing on their own.

6. Socializing and Adjourn.

Have fun. The idea of running a weight loss is supposed to be a benefit to the group leader as well. Have fun, make friends, and help others along the way.

CHAPTER 8

HOW TO RUN A WEIGHT LOSS GROUP

SUMMARY

- Starting a weight loss group may sound like a lot of work, but our helping of others helps us so much more in the long run.
- Have fun; get social!

APPENDIX:
KEEPING TRACK OF YOUR
MEASUREMENTS

The following tables have appeared previously in this book.
They appear here again to use for your records.

24-Hour Food Recall- Date:

Food Eaten	Amount	This Counts As

24-Hour Food Recall- Date:

Food Eaten	Amount	This Counts As
	252	

24-Hour Food Recall- Date:

Food Eaten	Amount	This Counts As

24-Hour Food Recall- Date:

Food Eaten	Amount	This Counts As
	253	

Personal Measurement Record:

Date				
Weight				
Neck Circumference				
Bust and/or Chest Circumference				
Waist Circumference				
Hip Circumference				
Sagittal Abdominal Height (stomach height in inches when laying down)				
Thigh Circumference				
Knee Circumference				
Calf Circumference				
Upper arm Circumference				
Lower arm Circumference				

ABOUT THE AUTHOR

Claudia Rachel Johnsen is a Ph.D. licensed nutritionist trained at the University of Connecticut Department of Nutrition, Tufts University Friedman School of Nutrition Science and Policy, and the Union Institute. This book is based on her original research.

www.ingramcontent.com/pod-product-compliance
Lightning Source LLC
Chambersburg PA
CBHW051436250726
48655CB00001B/84